NATURAL REMEDIES

Work with nature to protect your body and promote healing

pil

Publications International, Ltd.

Writers: Paul Bergner, Alexandra F. Griswold, Ph.D., David J. Hufford, Ph.D., Ara Der Marderosian, Ph.D., Bonnie O'Connor, Ph.D., Barbara Rieti, Ph.D., and Joan L. Saverino, Ph.D.

Images from Shutterstock.com and Wikipedia

ISBN: 978-1-64558-554-1

Manufactured in China.

8 7 6 5 4 3 2 1

Note: The editors of Publications International, Ltd., nor the authors, consultants, editors, or publisher take responsibility for any possible consequence from any treatment, procedure, exercise, dietary modification, action, or application of medication or preparation by any person reading or following the information in this book. The publication of this book does not constitute the practice of medicine, and this book does not attempt to replace your physician or your pharmacist. Before undertaking any course of treatment, the authors, consultants, editors, and publisher advise the reader to check with a physician or other health care provider.

Let's get social!

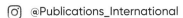 @Publications_International

@PublicationsInternational

www.pilbooks.com

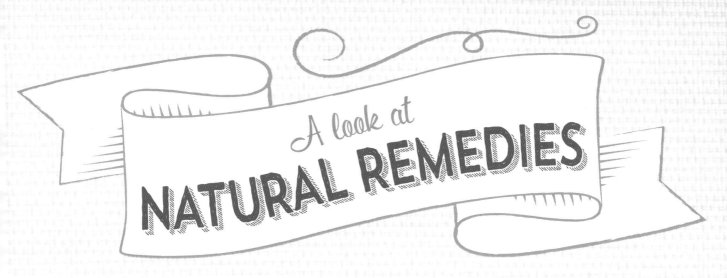

A look at NATURAL REMEDIES

Many people can respect nature—even during the most brutal blizzard or prolonged drought. However, many do not have the same respect for the remedies nature provides. The critical eyes of science have diminished the cultural relevance of natural remedies. But, in recent years, many people have begun to reconsider their attitudes toward the beneficial properties of nature. After all, even the experts can be wrong.

Natural remedies and beliefs in their efficacy are very closely related to peoples' experience with their bodies, their minds, and the world around them. No one is an expert on your experience except you! Ordinary people are sometimes wrong in ways that only an expert can best explain, but only the patient can decide what is right for them. Even if the doctor is right, the patient may not agree to the regimens of prescriptions, tests, and treatments proposed. Patients want to understand what is happening to them, why it is happening, and how they can treat it. But many times patients feel like their visits to the doctor's office are a one-way conversation in which the doctor glosses over the diagnoses and signs off on the prescriptions they need to take, confusing the patient more than helping them understand.

Today, more people are turning to natural remedies to treat their simple ailments and to garner a better understanding of their bodies and nature. They are beginning to balance the ways that they evaluate both scientific and natural remedies concerning their health. Many scientific studies are now verifying the effectiveness of natural remedies that have been used by many cultures for so long. But the science is still far behind understanding many of these remedies. Although clinical tests have been able to

3

identify certain chemical constituents and their ability to produce curative effects, many remedies have never been scientifically verified under the microscope. But just because it hasn't been verified, doesn't mean it wrong. And just because it has been verified, doesn't mean it's right for the patient.

NATURAL REMEDIES, "QUACKERY," AND THE HISTORY OF MEDICINE

Because of the great practical importance of medical beliefs and practices—both official and natural—we'll start with the related issues of efficacy, risk, and quackery. What reasons might we have to believe that some natural remedies "really work" and that some do not? Why is the word *quackery* often used in connection with folk traditions and their natural practices, and when is the term appropriate? What risks may be associated with using natural remedies?

Official medicine generally assumes that it has accepted, or is in the process of accepting, every healing practice that has been shown to be effective. Medical history has always been intimately associated with folk medicine and natural remedies, and today official medicine actually defines these medicines by exclusion. This very dominant position of official medicine, legally and in scientific terms, is a very new thing in Western culture. So we must begin with a little medical history.

Before the 20th century, the licensing of physicians was largely honorific, and it did not exclude unlicensed healers from practice. In 1760, New York City passed the first law for examining and exclusively licensing doctors, but that law was never enforced. In 1763, the physicians of Norwich, Connecticut, asked the colonial legislature for licensing "to distinguish between Honest and Ingenious physicians and the Quack or Empirical Pretender." The problem of competition was recognized as serious, but the request was denied. Following the American Revolution, medical societies organized and legislatures granted licensing, but these laws were powerless and ineffective. Americans have always been a fiercely independent lot, and the high value placed on individual choice was in direct conflict with the desire of medical professionals to control health care. As a result, a variety of popular forms of alternative medicines flourished openly. In fact, if we had been there in the mid-century, we would have had a hard time knowing just which practitioners were considered to be "regular" and which were "alternative."

Medical schools were, by and large, small businesses, and the quality of their graduates was very unreliable. Harvard was among the first of the to attempt reform. In 1869, Charles Eliot, the president of Harvard, said, "The ignorance and general incompetency of the average graduate of American Medical schools, at the time when he [is turned] loose upon the community, is something horrible to contemplate." Both the nature

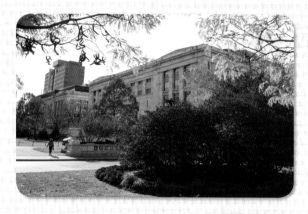

of the competition and the quality of medical education changed dramatically after Abraham Flexner, a young educator with a B.A. degree from Johns Hopkins, carried out a study of medical schools. His investigation was funded by the Carnegie Foundation for the Advancement of Teaching. Flexner made surprise visits to the schools and documented the often pathetic resources in laboratories, the lack of access to patients, the incompetent faculty, and the generally disreputable state of most American medical schools. His report, published in 1910, recommended that 100 of the 131 existing medical schools be closed, although 70 eventually survived. Flexner did not start the reform movement in medical education, but his report was a watershed event in the transformation of medicine. However, that reform not only improved the basics of education for "regular physicians," it also established a principle that many expected would eradicate the competition—including natural medicine. A whole new medicine, organized around "regular medicine" was to replace all separate medical sects.

The new medicine was to be objective and scientific. It was assumed that would mean that all treatments shown to work would be included and all those that were ineffective would be excluded. The Pure Food and Drug Act of 1906 and medical licensure soon consolidated the medical profession's political power. Using that power the profession actively worked to prevent others from practicing medicine without a license. Doctors labeled those who did not fit the medical model as "quacks," and their efforts to eradicate quackery were presented as public education and protection.

The word *quack* comes from the old Dutch word *quacksalver*. The term became popular in the 1500s and described people who sold salves and ointments—and who generally made exaggerated claims for them. Some have suggested that the word is also derived in part from *quicksilver*, which is the element mercury. Mercury was a common ingredient in regular medicines of the day as well as in the home remedies sold by quacks.

By the 20th century, the term quack was not at all restricted to ointment sellers. Modern dictionary definitions are very specific about what the word means: people who pretend to have medical knowledge that they do not in fact have. In other words, quackery is fraud. Unfortunately, the term is used very loosely, so that it is often applied to all sorts of healers whose practices were believed to be ineffective. The implication seems to be that any intelligent adult should know that if a type of healing is not offered by a licensed doctor, then it is useless and therefore must be fraud. This sloppy use of the word merely serves to insult those with whom conventional medicine disagrees. But still worse, it "gives cover" to the real medical frauds, of whom there are many. After all, with no distinction made between charlatans and sincere natural healers, it is much harder to identify the charlatans.

THE EFFECTIVENESS OF NATURAL MEDICINE

It has been shown that some natural remedies work—in the medical sense, that is. What's more, natural remedies are capable of serving goals that are broader and more complicated than those of modern medicine. Two compelling examples come from women's natural health traditions. For many years, women have learned from other women that eating live culture yogurt helps to reduce vaginal yeast infections. In 1992, a study published in the *Annals of Internal Medicine* concluded that this practice is, in fact, effective. Similarly, women's oral folk tradition has long taught that drinking cranberry juice can prevent and treat urinary tract infections. In 1994, a study published in the *Journal of the American Medical Association* concluded that this tradition is also correct—cranberry juice does have this effect.

Although there are prescription treatments available for both of these conditions, these natural remedies have the advantage of being inexpensive and without side effects. (They do not always work, however, and then prescription treatment may be necessary.) It is fascinating to consider that such widely known and practiced elements of natural medicine, used to treat very common medical problems, could have been ignored by conventional medicine for so long. Even now, after these studies, the use of these remedies has not become standard medical practice.

Prescription medications not only have their desired medical effects, but they also have side effects, some of which can be quite serious. The same is true for natural remedies. Many people have the mistaken idea that "If it's natural, it can't hurt me." Some of the most powerful poisons that we know of are found in nature. And every year, in addition to those individuals who are poisoned accidentally by plants, there are people who enter hospitals because plant remedies they prepared to treat medical conditions have in fact poisoned them. Poisoning can happen in several different ways.

Some plant medicines that are effective are simply too dangerous to use outside medical supervision. For example, the plant purple foxglove (*Digitalis purpurea*) contains digitalis, which has a powerful effect on the heart. Digitoxin and digoxin, the active ingredients of foxglove, have been used by physicians to treat some forms of heart disease since the 1920s. Digitalis was brought into medical use by William Withering, an English physician. He learned of the plant's use from an "old woman in Shropshire," an herbalist who had cured "dropsy" in individuals who doctors had given up on. (Dropsy is the accumulation of fluid in the body now known to be caused by congestive heart failure.) The Shropshire herbalist and other natural healers around the world had long used foxglove in this way, but the difference between a therapeutic dose and a toxic dose is very narrow and a poisonous overdose can be rapidly fatal. So, today, most herbalists recommend against using the plant outside of medical supervision. The plant leaf is still available, and some physicians are willing to prescribe it—as opposed to pills of synthetic digitalis or digoxin— for those who insist on natural treatment.

Foxglove

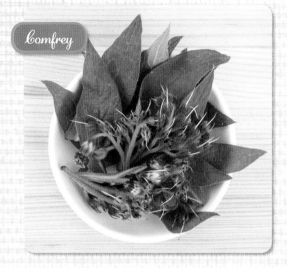

Comfrey

The deadly reaction to poisoning doesn't always occur quickly. Some popular plants in natural medicine have turned out to cause health problems when used over time. For example, comfrey is a plant that has been widely used as a medicine, but laboratory studies have shown that, with chronic use, it can lead to liver damage or even liver cancer. This kind of effect, something that develops slowly over time, is difficult for healers to recognize. Today, most herbalists and all medical authorities recommend against the internal use of comfrey.

A third way that plant medicines can become dangerous is through adulteration. This can happen either by accident or intentionally. Accidents happen when someone gathering herbs in the wild unintentionally picks the wrong plant or happens to grab two plants at once, one intended and the other not noticed. Also, many plants have poisonous parts that need to be separated from the edible or medicinal portions. Because many commercially available herbs come from outside the country and the products are not regulated, sometimes herbal medicines contain enough plant poison to cause sickness or even death. Even more alarming is the fact that some herbal medicines coming from outside the country have been found to have pharmaceutical drugs added to them. It seems that some marketers feel that these hidden drugs will improve sales by making the effects of the medicine more immediately noticeable.

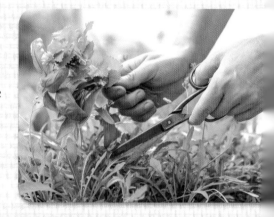

Either directly or through interaction with prescribed medication, such adulterated herbs can cause serious illness or death.

All three of these dangers are greatest for infants or very sick people with a low body weight. These dangers have been most frequently associated with commercially available herbal medicines. These risks are not enormous, but they are real. It seems prudent, therefore, to learn about plant medicine before you try herbal remedies. Watch for unexpected side effects and discontinue the herbal remedy if side effects occur. And, for infants, it would be wise in general to avoid the use of most herbal products.

NATURAL REMEDIES AND CULTURAL AUTHORITY

Natural remedies have long existed in tension with official medicine. An important source of that tension, and a large part of the difference between the two, involves cultural authority. Cultural authority is the power to make statements about how the world works—about the real nature of the world—and have those statements accepted. Throughout history, in most parts of the world, it was life

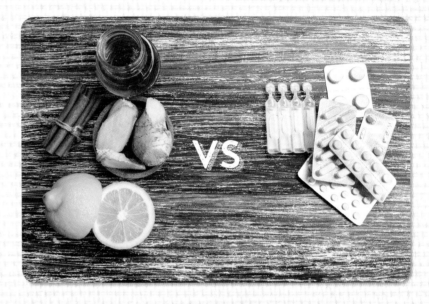

experience that gave people cultural authority. Religious status and a few other factors, such as the family into which a person was born, could also influence one's authority. In many natural medicine traditions, the knowledge of remedies is learned orally, representing the accumulated knowledge of past generations, and the evaluation of the treatment is done by the patient's observations of what seems to help.

In the 19th century, as science and technology began the rapid change that now characterizes our modern world, the structure of cultural authority changed. Scientific discoveries increasingly revealed important but invisible things about the world, from invisibly small bacteria to radiation. It became more and more obvious that we could not know everything important about the world with unaided senses. Too many things you could not see might make you sick. As a result of this growing division between everyday experience and scientific knowledge, which was strongly supported by the apparent advantages that technology could deliver, modern society shifted. An unspoken agreement developed in which the experts in science and technology were given cultural authority and the right to govern their own institutions.

The internal control of experts over the definition of their own expertise includes the opportunity to set the limits on the area to which their expertise applies. The result is that the scope of expert cultural authority has grown consistently in modern society. Of course, that means that, at the same time, the scope of authority based on life experience, and not technical training, has decreased. The best medical care has come to be understood not as the accumulation of past wisdom but rather as the very latest technique, and the very latest technique is often explained in terms of how it puts past ideas to rest. Very recent training has largely replaced, in the minds of many, the value of lifelong clinical experience. In this modern view, elders are people who require extra care, not people you turn to for an understanding of the world. And as far as a patient's right to evaluate his own treatment, the double-blind, placebo-controlled clinical trial has been developed. The patient's ability to know what really helps has been discredited as "merely subjective."

Up through the 1960s many believed that this social change in authority was irreversible and that technical knowledge would become the only kind of knowledge considered valid. But the 1960s brought deep change—ranging from the Hippie movement to the consumer movement, civil rights and women's liberation, even the Charismatic movement in Christian religion. All of these changes were rebellion against various kinds of authority and were a reassertion of the right of people to find, in their own experience, some valid basis for un-

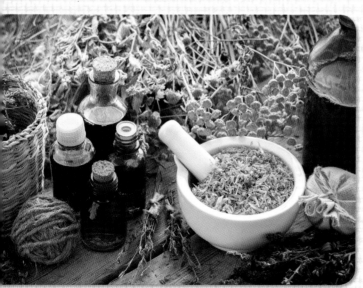

derstanding and evaluating the world. The result has not been the complete overthrow of expert authority, but rather a process of trimming that authority back. In medicine, the idea of "informed consent," which requires doctors to tell patients what is proposed as treatment and why it is proposed, is an example of the reduction of medical authority and the return of some authority to the patient.

Natural medicine is made up of traditions in which the wisdom of past generations is gathered. Therefore, the idea that natural medicine contains important knowledge, some of which may have been forgotten in modern times, depends on a recognition of the value of life experience and the possibility that people really knew something—even before there were microscopes and X-ray machines. This idea is receiving renewed interest, thanks to the recent changes in cultural authority.

Ideally our society will find a balance on these issues. There is no need to decide between life experience and technical training, or between official medicine and natural medicine. Both seem to have great value. The greatest value will come from being able to understand what is appropriate to each. Herbal treatments clearly have some value, but they also have risks. The sense of closeness to nature and the avoidance of harsh side effects, which can come from the proper use of herbs, are best evaluated on the basis of life experience. Only the patient can answer: "How do these herbs make me feel?" and "How much did the side effects of the remedy bother me?" On the other hand, many serious illnesses require medical expertise for their successful management. Some patients believe they can increase the success of their medical treatment by also using natural remedies. This is a good idea, as long as there is an informed process in which both the doctor and the patient understand the treatments being used.

NATURAL REMEDIES AND ALTERNATIVE MEDICINE

As the modern understanding of authority and life experience have improved in recent decades, we have also become aware that natural remedies have persisted, adapted, and grown. They have shared in the social processes by which alternative medicine has become so enormously popular.

The definition developed by the 1995 Complementary and Alternative Medicine Research Methodology Conference, sponsored by the NIH Office of Alternative Medicine, identifies alternative medicine as all health ideas and practices at any particular time in history or in any society that are different from those found in official medicine. Obviously, then, these natural remedies are a kind of alternative medicine.

We can refer to many forms of alternative medicine as "cosmopolitan," meaning that they are present in many different regions and are similar wherever they are found. All of conventional medicine and much of alternative medicine in the United States consists of cosmopolitan traditions. Homeopathy and chiropractic, two prominent alternative examples, each depends heavily on print— from professional journals to textbooks to popular works read by the public.

Cosmopolitan alternative systems tend to stay the same in very different places because print media has a conservative influence on the tradition. This influence is partly due to the formal institutions that maintain the use of print: chiropractic colleges, homeopathic institutes, certification, the development of a standard "canon" of published works. In turn, these formal institutions make it easier for cosmopolitan systems to generate a commercial base, from cash fees for service to insurance reimbursement. The resources that become available with a commercial base facilitate the use of print and electronic media, the development of formal institutions, and so forth.

Some natural remedy traditions have retained many ideas for centuries, but other elements of them have changed very rapidly. This combination makes natural remedies very adaptable, and this is what accounts for its regional variation.

Most alternative medicine traditions stress the underlying causes of disease as well as the immediate causes. The underlying causes are usually seen as some kind of imbalance or lack of harmony within the body. The techniques of natural medicine are almost entirely ones that are broadly legal, require little or no technology, and are therefore available to practically everyone. Although the highly learned healer generally has a body of knowledge that requires time and special circumstances to acquire, the individual elements are nonetheless generally available to all. Thus, the materials of these systems can readily be organized into all levels of health behavior—from first aid and home treatment to the most specialized and authoritative forms. This makes it very easy for people to enter natural medical systems. Natural medicine lacks many of the official barriers found in scientific medicine, and it makes available to patients a wide range of options for varying levels of personal involvement and decision making.

For many patients, this is an attractive feature of natural medicine. In the pages to come you will find a great variety of natural medical practices. Some of these practices will seem simple, such as drinking cranberry juice to reduce the risk of urinary tract infections. Others will seem a little farfetched. The remedies described in this book come from many different communities and represent the accumulated ideas and observations of centuries of healers. Like scientific medicine, some natural medicine is obsolete, some is dangerous, and some is ahead of its time. But all of these ideas represent the struggles of human communities to make sense of disease, suffering, and death and to do something about the human condition.

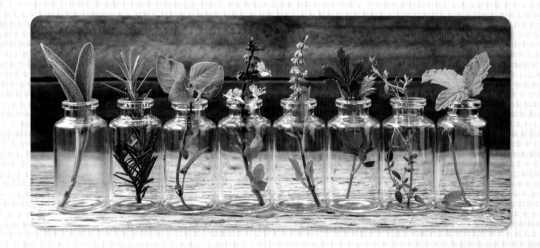

A Look at Natural Remedies

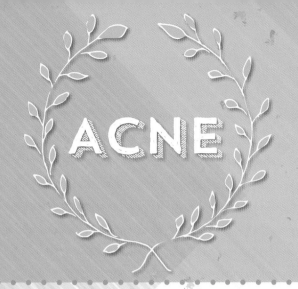

ACNE

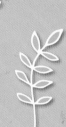

Although these natural remedies date back centuries, they have proven time and again that they have what it takes when it comes to treating acne.

Acne often begins with the normal hormonal changes of puberty. The hormone testosterone increases at that time in both men and women and causes an increase in the size and secretions of the sebaceous glands in the skin that produce sebum (an oily secretion). Most excess oil produced by these glands leaves the skin through the hair follicles (the tubelike structures from which hairs develop). Sometimes, however, oil clogs these tubes and creates comedones (blocked hair follicles). Comedones are what form the initial bumps of acne.

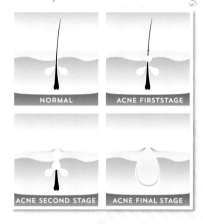

If comedones are open to the surface of the skin, they are called blackheads. They contain sebum from the sebaceous glands, bacteria, and any skin tissue that accumulates near the surface. Comedones that are closed at the surface are called whiteheads.

Plugged hair follicles can rupture internally, resulting in a discharge of their contents into the surrounding tissues. Bacteria in the injured area can sometimes lead to more widespread inflammation and the formation of painful cysts. In severe cases, pitting and scarring result.

Acne normally resolves all by itself without specific medical treatment. For some individuals, however, acne can continue into the adult years. In women, acne may cycle with the menses, due to varying output of hormones. Oily cosmetics or moisturizers can sometimes cause acne or make an existing case worse. And although a link has not been medically proven, many people notice acne flare-ups when they're under stress. There is, however, no medical evidence to suggest that what you eat affects acne.

Acne has no prevention or cure, but there are several treatments. The main treatment for mild acne is thorough cleansing with a mild soap two to three times a day. Some over-the-counter medications, particularly lotions or creams containing benzoyl peroxide, can help troubled skin as well. For persistent acne, a doctor might prescribe an antibiotic preparation that can be applied to the surface of the skin or an oral antibiotic, such as tetracycline. Antibiotics do not heal the pimples or prevent their formation, but they do prevent their infection or rupture, and subsequent inflammation of the surrounding tissues. Thus, antibiotics may also help to prevent scarring. Unfortunately, oral antibiotics can also kill the friendly bacteria in the intestinal tract and cause unpleasant digestive side effects, such as gas, bloating, and indigestion. Antibiotics may also promote intestinal or vaginal yeast infections.

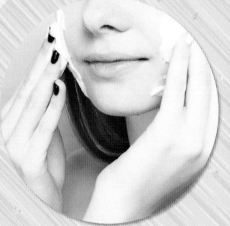

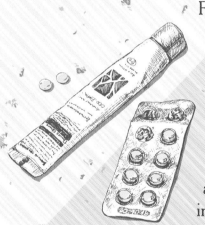

For severe acne, the drug isotretinoin may be prescribed. This drug works by temporarily suppressing the production of secretions by the sebaceous glands. This drug can have very serious side effects and should never be used without the supervision of a doctor. In fact, for patients taking isotretinoin, standard medical practice is to run routine blood and liver function tests each month to see if the drug is damaging the liver. In addition, isotretinoin should not be used by any woman who is—or who thinks she may be—pregnant. Use of this drug in any amount for even short periods during pregnancy is associated with an extremely high risk of birth defects.

Trying vitamin supplementation might make a prudent first course of action before trying prescription medications. Supplementation with zinc, for example, is one scientifically validated nutritional treatment of acne. (Some acne patients have lowered serum and tissue levels of zinc.) A 1989 double-blind clinical trial showed that zinc supplementation significantly improved the acne of the participants in the study.

Although the natural remedies that follow date back centuries, they have proven time and again that they have what it takes when it comes to treating acne.

Acne

REMEDIES FOR ACNE

Clay Packs

Many remedies call for the use of astringent washes and poultices. These remedies naturally absorb or "draw" the excess oily secretions out of the skin. Applying clay packs to the face is a popular acne remedy among today's Seventh Day Adventists, a religious movement that uses many natural remedies. (This remedy was also used by German immigrants at the turn of the century.) Today, you can purchase cosmetic grade clay for the same purpose.

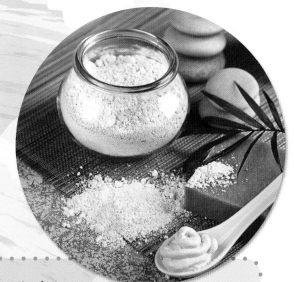

Directions: Using bentonite clay or other cosmetic clay, mix the clay into one cup of warm (not hot) water until it is the consistency of a thick pea soup. Apply it to the skin. Let it stay on for at least forty minutes—several hours if possible. Wipe off using water and a wash cloth. You may need to scrub with the cloth if the clay has dried completely—but don't scrub your skin too hard! Wipe the clay off over a bowl and discard the dry clay in your garden or on your lawn. (Clay can accumulate and stop up your plumbing pipes.) Repeat as often as desired.

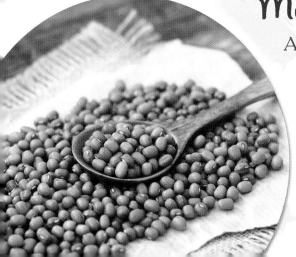

Mung Beans

A Chinese remedy for acne is to apply a paste of mung beans to the face. The astringent properties of the beans draw the oil out of the skin.

Directions: Use a coffee grinder to grind the dry mung beans to a powder. Mix with warm water and follow the instructions above for applying a clay mask.

Canaigre

Traditional Hispanic residents of the American Southwest use the herb canaigre (*Rumex hymenosepalus*) as a poultice to draw oil from the skin. Canaigre contains high amounts of tannin, which acts as an astringent.

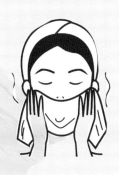

Directions: Chop or grind one ounce of the root, and simmer in two quarts of water for twenty minutes. Soak a cloth in the tea and apply it hot to the face for ten to fifteen minutes. Save the tea to reheat for future use. Apply the poultice once or twice a day until skin improves and complexion clears.

Burdock

Burdock tea has been used to treat acne throughout the eastern states and at least as far west as Indiana. Burdock (*Arctium lappa*) is slightly diaphoretic, which means it brings blood circulation to the surface of the skin to promote sweating. The increased local circulation of immune elements of the blood may help fight the infection and inflammation of acne. Burdock also contains a high amount of starch, and, applied locally, the starch may help absorb excess oils from the skin.

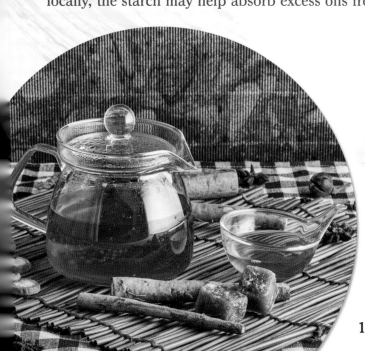

Directions: To make a cup of burdock tea, take one ounce of the ground dried root and simmer it in two quarts of water for twenty minutes. Strain (saving the root) and drink three to four cups a day. You can also apply a poultice to the affected area. After making the tea, wrap up the leftover root in a cloth. Moisten both the cloth and the root with a little of the hot tea. Apply for fifteen to twenty minutes. Do this as often as desired. Continue using until complexion clears.

Acne

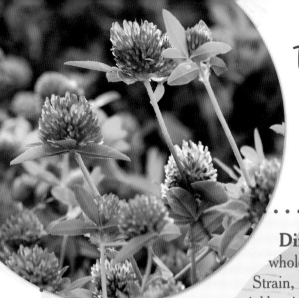

Red Clover

Indiana farmers today still utilize a poultice of red clover plants as a treatment for acne. Red clover (*Trifolium pratense*) contains several constituents that may thin the oily secretions of the face, making the oil easier to remove.

Directions: Using just enough water to cover, simmer whole flowering red clover plants in a pot until tender. Strain, press the plants into a thick mass, and sprinkle with white flour. (The flour helps add consistency to the poultice and will help to draw the oils from the skin.) Place the poultice directly on the skin. Leave on for half an hour. You can use the red clover poultice several times a day. This poultice can last a few days if it's kept in the refrigerator between applications.

Stinging Nettle

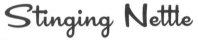

Drinking a tea of stinging nettle (*Urtica dioica*) is a Romani remedy for treating acne. You can also apply stinging nettle tea as a face wash. Nettle is astringent and drying and may help reduce the oily secretions of the skin.

Directions: Place one ounce of dried stinging nettle leaf in a one-quart canning jar. Fill the jar with boiling water. Cover and let sit overnight or until the water reaches room temperature. Drink two to three cups a day. You can also reheat a portion of the tea and apply it to the face as a warm wash once or twice a day. Handle carefully to avoid the plant's stinging hairs.

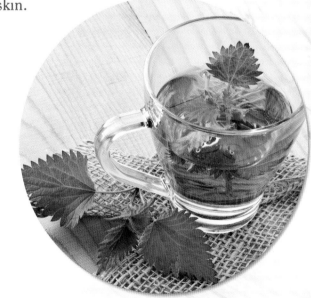

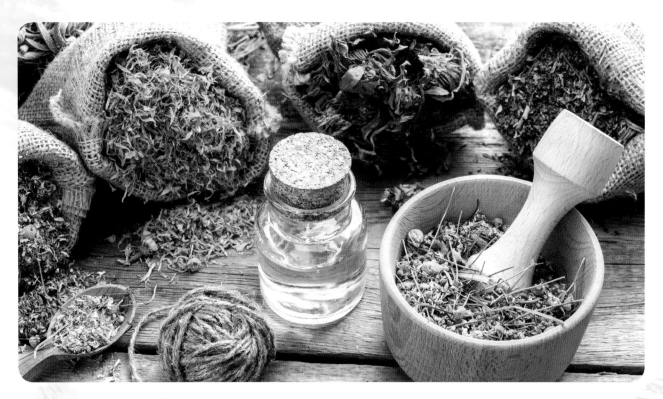

Essential Oils

The Winnebago Indians of the last century treated acne by making a poultice of the boiled leaves of the wild bergamot plant (*Monarda fistulosa*). Besides the oil-absorbing properties of the leaves, the essential oils of the plant are drying and antibacterial. This plant is probably not available in your local store, but common thyme (*Thymus vulgaris*) or its essential oil may be substituted. Essential oils are available where aromatherapy products are sold. Both wild bergamot and thyme contain the volatile oil thymol, which has mild antibacterial properties.

Other essential oils used as natural remedies for acne include the oils of juniper, thyme, and rose. If you decide to use essential oils, be sure to dilute them with alcohol or glycerin before applying them to the skin, however. Some pure concentrated oils can cause second- and third-degree skin burns if left in place for too long.

Directions: Use a pleasant carrier oil or cream such as almond oil or cold cream. Use six to eight drops of the concentrated oil for each ounce of the carrier. Mix well and apply to the face. Wipe off after twenty minutes. Apply once a day. Continue to use until skin improves. Avoid the eye area.

Acne

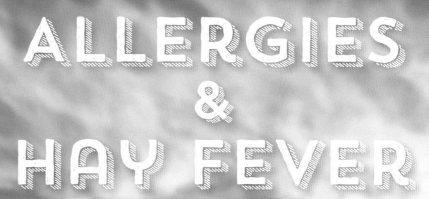

ALLERGIES & HAY FEVER

For millions of Americans, each change of season brings its own brand of allergies and irritants—and a variety of natural remedies.

Our bodies are constantly assaulted by substances from the environment, in the form of bacteria, viruses, molds, dust, pollen, and other potential invaders. Our immune system reacts to these substances through chemical and blood responses that attempt to neutralize the invaders or eliminate them from the body. One specialized immune response is the allergic reaction, in which specialized cells stimulated by an invading substance release the chemical histamine into the tissues. The histamine can cause swelling, increased circulation, and sneezing, actions designed to isolate the invader, eliminate it, or render it harmless. An allergic reaction can occur in the respiratory tract, skin, or eyes.

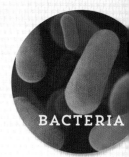

An allergic reaction is a healthy, protective response to an invader, but, in some individuals, the body overreacts, and the uncomfortable reactions are far in excess of what is necessary to neutralize the offending substance. The most noticeable allergic symptoms are sneezing, red swollen eyes, shortness of breath (in asthma), rashes, eczema, or the swelling that accompanies insect bites and stings. Food allergies can also cause symptoms in the digestive tract, but these are usually less noticeable to the sufferer than the external reactions above. The worst type of allergic reaction—called anaphylaxis—is an overwhelming allergic reaction that can lead to death. Any swelling of the airways or shortness of breath during an allergic reaction is an emergency.

Allergies tend to run in families, so some people may be genetically predisposed to having them. It has also been suggested that nutrient deficiencies common in the modern diet may also contribute to allergies. Dietary deficiencies of calcium and magnesium, which are common deficiencies in Americans, can also increase allergic symptoms. Studies have shown that the body's stores of vitamin C correlate inversely with the release of histamine during an allergy attack, so an abundant dietary intake of vitamin C may reduce allergy symptoms. Omega-3 essential fatty acids, such as those that occur naturally in cold-water fish and wild game, are also natural anti-inflammatory substances that can reduce the intensity of allergies.

Antihistamine drugs and avoidance of allergens are the most common conventional treatments for symptoms of allergy. The drugs work by blocking the effects of histamine in the tissues, but they do not reduce its release. Desensitization involves medical treatments where small amounts of an allergen may also be injected into the body in the form of allergy shots in order to reduce the body's reaction to it. The folk remedies listed here do not address the cause of allergies but may reduce allergy symptoms through their astringent or anti-inflammatory actions.

BACTERIA

VIRUS

MOLD

POLLEN

REMEDIES FOR ALLERGIES & HAY FEVER

HORSERADISH

Horseradish (*Armoracia rusticana*), popular today as a sushi condiment, was an early American remedy for hay fever. If you've used it as a condiment, you're probably well aware that it causes watery eyes and a burning sensation in the sinus tissues. These effects are due to its constituent allyl-isothiocyanate, which is related chemically to the substances in watercress, red radish, and brown and yellow mustard. Scientific studies have shown that allyl-isothiocyanate has decongestant and antiasthmatic properties.

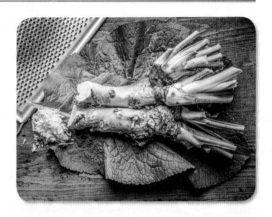

Directions: Purchase grated horseradish as a condiment. Take a dose of ¼ teaspoon during a congestive hay fever attack. You can take horseradish as often as desired—or as much as you can stand!

An alternate method, if you have access to fresh horseradish root, comes from an old New England remedy. Take fresh horseradish roots, wash, and blend, skin and all, in your blender. Fill half of a one-quart jar with the ground roots. Add enough vinegar to cover the roots, and close the jar tightly. Store the jar at room temperature. When suffering a hay fever attack, remove the cap, place your nose into the jar, and sniff or inhale. (Do this carefully at first to avoid irritating your nose and eyes.) Quickly replace the cap to keep the remaining aromatic substances from escaping. This treatment requires fresh-ground horseradish; most likely, it will lose its potency after four or five days.

HORSEMINT

In the medicine of southern Appalachia, horsemint (*Monarda punctata*) is a traditional treatment for hay fever. Horsemint may be inhaled, or you can drink it as a simple tea. Horsemint is not readily available in stores today, but its anti-allergic constituent is probably the essential oil thymol. Scientific studies have shown that thymol reduces swelling in the bronchial tract, relaxes the trachea, and acts as an anti-inflammatory and mild antibacterial. The kitchen spice thyme also contains large amounts of this aromatic oil and can be substituted for horsemint.

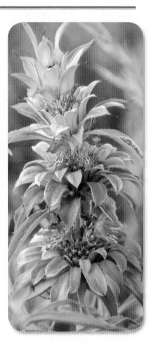

Directions: Place ½ ounce of ground thyme in a one-pint jar and cover with boiling water. Close the jar tightly and let the mixture cool for half an hour. Remove the lid and inhale, taking a few deep breaths. Do this as needed throughout the day.

CHAMOMILE & THYME OIL

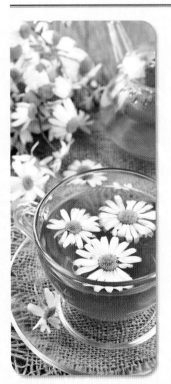

German immigrants inhaled the fumes of chamomile tea (*Matricaria recutita*) to treat bouts of hay fever. In contemporary German naturopathic medicine, three to five drops of the essential oil of thyme is added to chamomile tea for the same purpose. (The action of thyme oil is described under the remedy Horsemint.) Chamomile contains the essential oil azulene and related oils that are anti-inflammatory and anti-allergic, as well as the oil alpha-bisabolol, which is also an anti-inflammatory.

Directions: Place ½ ounce of chamomile flowers in a one-quart jar. Fill two thirds of the jar with boiling water. Add three to five drops of essential oil of thyme. Cover and let cool for half an hour. Open the lid and inhale the fumes, taking a few deep breaths. Repeat as desired throughout the day. (Be careful of inhaling flower dust, because the pollen causes allergies in some people.)

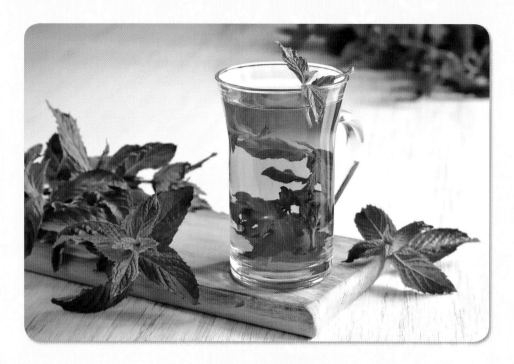

MINT TEAS

Inhaling, drinking, or washing affected skin areas with mint teas can be accredited in this country to the natural medicine of the Seneca Indians. The plants used to make the teas are peppermint (*Mentha piperita*) and spearmint (*Mentha spicata*). In China, cornmint (*Mentha arvensis*), which is similar in its chemical composition to peppermint, is used. (Mint teas have been used to treat allergies in China at least since the 7th century AD).

When consumed as a tea or inhaled, the essential oils in the mints act as a decongestant. When applied to the skin, the menthol in peppermint and cornmint produces a cooling sensation and reduces itching. (Spearmint contains little menthol, however, so it does not have this effect on the skin.) All three of the mints contain other anti-inflammatory and mild antibacterial constituents.

Directions: Place ½ ounce of dried mint leaves in a one-quart jar. Fill two thirds of the jar with boiling water and cover the jar tightly. Let cool for half an hour. Strain and drink. The tea's fumes will also help relieve congestion.

EYEBRIGHT

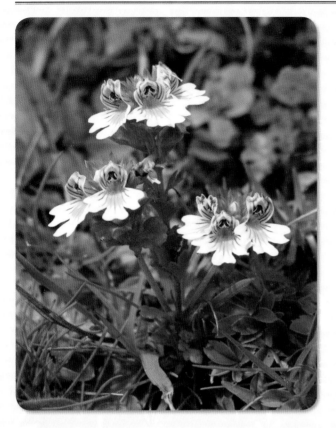

The use of eyebright (*Euphrasia officinalis*) to treat allergies in the eastern United States dates back at least 150 years and may have had its roots among German immigrants. At the turn of the century, Eclectic physicians, a group of M.D.s who used mostly herbs as medicines, also used eyebright to treat allergy symptoms among their patients. During the same period, the pharmaceutical companies Parke Davis and Eli Lilly sold eyebright allergy preparations to the public. Eyebright is still used today in Appalachia as a natural remedy for allergies.

Eyebright contains the constituents caffeic acid and ferulic acid, both of which have an anti-inflammatory effect. The caffeic acid also has specific antihistamine effects.

Directions: You can purchase eyebright tincture in a health food store or herb shop. Take a dropperful every three to four hours during the height of allergy season.

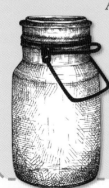

Another option is to make your own tincture. Place two ounces of dried eyebright leaves in a one-pint jar and fill the jar with grain alcohol or 100 proof gin or vodka. Cover the jar and let it stand in a cool, dark place for three weeks, shaking the jar each day. After three weeks, strain and store the solution in the refrigerator. Take as directed above.

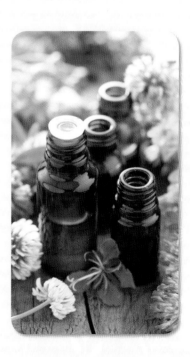

ANXIETY & NERVOUSNESS

Probably no single situation or condition causes anxiety disorders. Rather, physical and environmental triggers may combine to create a particular anxiety illness.

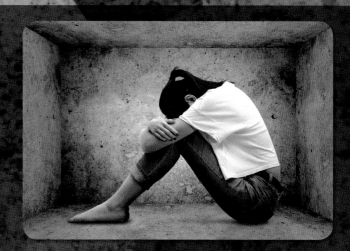

Everyone experiences some anxiety. Anxiety helps us stay alert and adapt to the ever-changing demands of our environment. Anxiety is really the body's "early warning system" against harm. When we feel danger, the alarm goes off to warn us and prevent injury. The body responds immediately to the alarm emotionally, physically, and behaviorally. Emotionally, we may feel fear, doom, or anger. Physically, our hearts race, muscles tense, breathing becomes rapid, and palms and feet start to sweat. We respond behaviorally by getting ready to fight or flee from danger.

The anxiety warning system works fine when there's clear and present danger, but anxiety can become a problem for people when they perceive harmless situations as threatening.

There is no single reason why some people experience episodes of chronic anxiety. Some of these individuals will benefit from visiting a psychotherapist, who can help them sort out internal conflicts or past conditioning that may be causing the emotional state. Any physical change, such as illness, can also cause anxiety. Anemia, diabetes, premenstrual syndrome, menopause, thyroid disorder, hypoglycemia, pulmonary disease, endocrine tumors, and other conditions can cause anxiety symptoms. Other individuals simply need to improve their nutrition and lifestyle—anxiety can be the symptom of several nutrient deficiencies or lifestyle habits that are common in modern society.

One of the most commonly overlooked causes of anxiety and nervousness in modern life is related to caffeine consumption. Even moderate amounts of caffeine can create nervous symptoms severe enough to earn a diagnosis of chronic anxiety—and a subsequent prescription of sedative drugs or referral to a therapist.

You don't need to take a lot of caffeine in order to experience these symptoms. Some of us can get away with drinking a few cups of coffee every day, but others can develop the symptoms of caffeinism even from a small amount. In one scientific study, patients with anxiety disorder rated their symptoms on a standard test. Their levels of anxiety and depression correlated directly with the amount of caffeine they consumed. In another study, a group of six anxiety patients who consumed the caffeine equivalent of one to three cups of coffee—about the average daily intake for Americans—cut their intake to zero. Within twelve to eighteen months, five of the six patients no longer experienced symptoms of anxiety.

One scientific theory suggests that anxiety is closely associated with the balance of the substances lactate and pyruvate in the body. These two substances are associated with energy production within the cells, and high lactate levels may cause anxiety. Alcohol, caffeine, and sugar all increase lactate levels, and the B-vitamins niacin and thiamine and the mineral magnesium all lower it. Deficiencies of the B-vitamins as well as omega-3 fatty acids, such as occur naturally in fish and wild game, may thus contribute to anxiety.

Conventional treatment of anxiety is primarily with drugs of the benzodiazepine class, such as Valium and Xanax. Anxiety patients are often treated by psychotherapists as well. Here are some natural remedies you can try to help ease feelings of stress and anxiety.

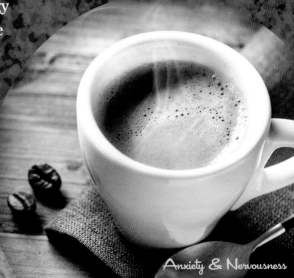

Anxiety & Nervousness

Remedies for
Anxiety & Nervousness

Valerian

In natural medicine traditions, valerian is considered a universal sedative. The Greeks used valerian as a relaxant and antispasmodic. The herb was also used in the medicine of India and Japan. Today, Mexicans and Mexican-Americans use varieties of the plant native to their regions. An African-American remedy from Louisiana is to put valerian root in a pillow and inhale its fragrance as you sleep. Valerian continues to be used as a sedative among today's Appalachians as well.

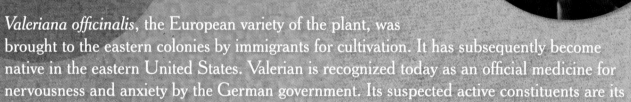

Valeriana officinalis, the European variety of the plant, was brought to the eastern colonies by immigrants for cultivation. It has subsequently become native in the eastern United States. Valerian is recognized today as an official medicine for nervousness and anxiety by the German government. Its suspected active constituents are its

Valerian-Hop Tea

German immigrants of the late 18th century treated nervousness with a mixture of equal portions of valerian (*Valeriana officinalis*) and hop (*Humulus lupulus*). Commercial combinations of these two herbs are still popular in Germany today. Hop has also been used as a sedative among British immigrants, Seventh Day Adventists, Indiana farmers, and residents of the American Southwest.

Directions: Mix equal amounts by volume of dried and chopped valerian root and hop in a bowl. Place one tablespoon of the mixture in a cup and fill the cup with boiling water. Cover the cup and let stand for twenty minutes. Strain and drink three cups a day. Take nightly for up to three weeks.

essential oils. Valerian has proven to be as effective as the sedative Valium in some clinical trials, although it has no relationship chemically to that drug. Valerian can cause stimulation rather than sedation in some individuals, however, especially those with "hot" constitutions, as might be indicated by feelings of warmth, by red flushed cheeks, and by desire for cool drinks.

According to Chinese medicine, this strong "fire-type" personality should avoid alcohol and stimulating foods and, instead, balance their excess heat with cooling foods and calming herbs. Heating herbs such as valerian increase circulation, which is already excessive in those with a hot nature.

Directions: Place two to three teaspoons of dried chopped valerian root in a cup and cover with boiling water. Cover the cup and let stand for fifteen minutes. Drink two to three cups a day for up to three weeks. Individuals who use valerian for longer than three weeks, or who use valerian to help them get to sleep, can ultimately develop lethargy or hangover effects.

Here is a recipe from Romani medicine for valerian wine: Take two handfuls of chopped valerian root, one whole clove, one orange rind, one sprig of rosemary, and one quart of dry white wine. Place the dried herbs in a one-quart jar and cover with the wine. Seal the container and allow to stand in a cool dark place for one cycle of the moon. Strain and store. Take one tablespoon of the mixture three times a day for up to three weeks. Note: valerian has a disagreeable odor.

Catnip

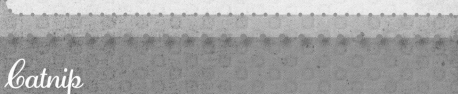

Catnip tea has been used as a popular sleep aid in America since the arrival of European immigrants in New England. The popularity of the tea spread rapidly in the New World, and American Indians soon adopted its use. The Onondaga and Cayuga Indian tribes used it to calm restless children, and European New Englanders gave it to adults for nervous disorders, including nervous breakdown. Today, catnip remains a common natural remedy among residents of Appalachia.

Directions: Place one to three teaspoons of the dried herb in a cup and cover with boiling water. Cover the cup and let stand for ten minutes. Strain and drink three cups a day. Use as needed.

Skullcap

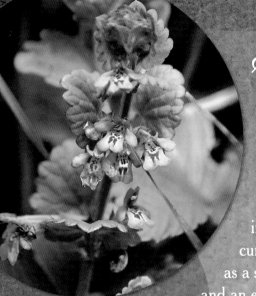

More than a hundred species of skullcap (*Scutellaria* spp.) grow throughout the world. North American varieties of the herb were used by American Indian tribes such as the Penobscot, Iroquois, and Cherokee to treat diarrhea and heart disease and to promote menstruation and eliminate afterbirth. Skullcap received its common name, mad dog weed, in the 18th century, when the herb was widely prescribed as a cure for rabies. It is still used today in Appalachian folk medicine as a sedative. The suspected medicinal constituents are flavonoids and an essential oil.

Directions: Put two teaspoonfuls of dried skullcap leaves in a cup and fill with boiling water. Cover and steep for fifteen minutes. Strain and drink three to four cups a day as needed.

Rosemary

European and Spanish immigrants brought the herb rosemary (*Rosmarinus officinalis*) with them to cultivate in the New World. Rosemary was later used by early Californians to rid the body of "evil spirits" or to treat epilepsy, which in ancient times was considered to be a form of possession.

Rosemary has long been used in European and Chinese medicine to calm the nerves. Medical experts in the United States continue to recommend rosemary to treat nervous conditions. Rosemary's analgesic and antispasmodic properties are also recognized by the German government; the herb is used there as an official medical treatment for spastic conditions, including epilepsy.

Directions: Add one or two teaspoons of the dried herb to a cup and fill the cup with boiling water. Cover the cup and let stand ten minutes. Strain and drink two to three cups a day as needed.

Vervain

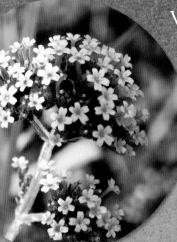

Vervain (*Verbena* spp.) has long been used as a sedative among residents of the Southwest and Appalachia. It has been used in European medicine since antiquity for the same purposes. Its constituent verbenalin promotes relaxation. Vervain is claimed to be especially useful for recovery from the exhaustion of long-term stress.

Directions: Add one or two teaspoons of the dried herb to a cup and fill with boiling water. Cover the cup and let stand ten minutes. Strain and drink two to three cups a day as needed.

Passion Flower

Of nineteen passion flower species worldwide, eight have been used as sedatives by various cultures. Passion flower (*Passiflora incarnata*) is native from Florida to Texas and may also be found as far north as Missouri. The herb is abundant in South America; it's long-time use as a sedative there is recorded in Brazilian medicine.

The passion flower species *P. incarnata* was introduced into American professional medicine in 1840 after medical doctors in Mississippi experimented with it and demonstrated its sedative effects. Thereafter the herb was mainly used by doctors of the Eclectic school. Passion flower is still popularly used as a sedative among residents of southern Appalachia and among the Amish. The herb is also widely cultivated in Europe for medicinal purposes; it is approved by the German government as a sedative medicine. Passion flower is a gentle sedative and is often combined with other plants. Most likely, its active constituent is an alkaloid, called passiflorine (or harmane).

Directions: Place one heaping teaspoon of dried passion flower in a cup, fill the cup with boiling water, cover, and steep ten minutes. Strain and drink as needed.

Motherwort

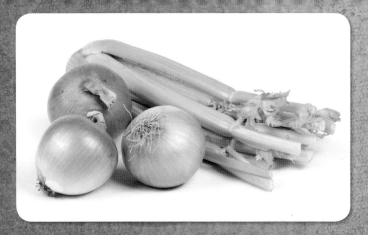

Motherwort is a mild relaxing agent often recommended by herbalists to reduce anxiety and depression and treat nervousness, insomnia, heart palpitations, and rapid heart rate. Motherwort (*Leonurus cardiaca*) has been used in Europe since antiquity as a sedative and to treat menstrual irregularities. It probably came to North America with physicians among the British colonists. American Indian tribes later adopted the herb's medicinal uses.

Today, in Germany, motherwort is an approved medicine for treating anxiety. It is also used in contemporary Chinese medicine for the same purpose. The herb contains a chemical called leonurine, which may encourage uterine contractions, however. Thus, you will want to avoid motherwort if you are pregnant or trying to conceive a child.

Directions: Place one to two teaspoons of motherwort herb in a cup and fill the cup with boiling water. Cover the cup and let stand for ten to fifteen minutes. Strain and drink. The tea's taste is bitter. Don't drink more than two to three cups a day.

Celery-Onion Salad

Some contemporary Indiana residents, according to a survey of recorded natural remedies used in the state, suggested eating celery and onions to overcome nervousness. Both celery and onions contain large amounts of potassium and folic acid. Studies have

Asafoetida

Asafoetida (*Ferula assafoetida*), a relative of garlic and onions, is a traditional medicine from Asia. Its usage as a calming agent probably arrived in North America by way of immigrating European physicians. The Eclectic physicians of the 1920s used asafoetida as a sedative. The herb is still used today in Appalachian herbalism to treat nervousness and mental stress.

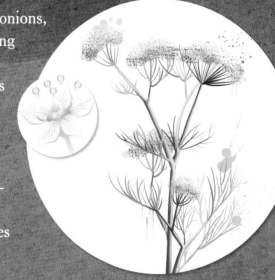

Asafoetida has at least two sedative constituents, including ferulic acid, which is analgesic, antispasmodic, and acts as a muscle relaxant, and valeric acid, which induces sleep, relaxes muscle, and acts as a sedative.

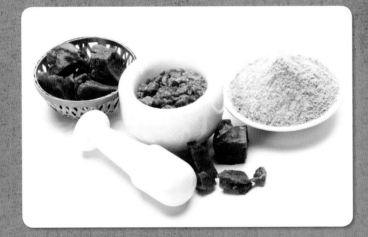

Directions: Stir ¼ teaspoon of asafoetida powder into a little warm water and drink. Do this two or three times a day. If asafoetida begins to cause heartburn, reduce the dose or try another sedative. Asafoetida has a strong, disagreeable garlic-like odor.

shown that deficiencies of each of these nutrients can cause fatigue, insomnia, and nervousness.

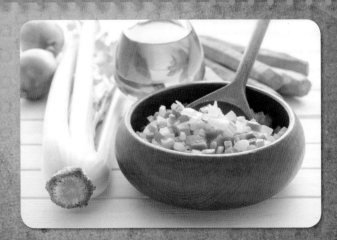

Directions: Eat two cups of either celery or onions, or a combination of the two, raw or cooked, with each meal for a week or two.

33

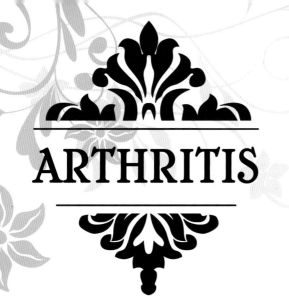

ARTHRITIS

Millions of Americans are caught in the grip of a form of arthritis or rheumatic disease. While there are no cures, there are natural remedies you can try to help ease discomfort.

In a nutshell, arthritis means "inflammation of the joints." Rheumatism is an old medical term that was used to describe inflammation of either joints or muscles. Rheum was thought to be a watery mucus-like secretion, sometimes brought on by cold weather. Joint or muscle pain was thought to be caused by such secretions trapped in the tissues. Although the concept is not far from the truth—inflammation is usually accompanied by swelling and a build-up of fluid—the modern explanation of arthritis is much more precise.

Today's medical experts suggest there are at least twenty-three varieties of arthritis, including rheumatoid arthritis and osteoarthritis, the two most common types. With osteoarthritis—sometimes called degenerative joint disease, or DJD—there is a gradual wearing away of cartilage in the joints. Healthy cartilage is the elastic tissue that lines and cushions the joints and allows bones to move smoothly against one another. When this cartilage deteriorates, the bones rub together, causing pain and swelling. Permanent damage and stiffness of the joints is possible.

Rheumatoid arthritis can attack at any age. This form of arthritis affects all the connective tissues, as well as other organs. The precise cause of rheumatoid arthritis is unknown. Some researchers believe that a virus triggers the disease, causing an auto-immune response whereby the body attacks it own tissues. However, evidence for this theory is inconclusive. What is confirmed is the progression of the condition. First, the synovium (the thin membrane that lines and lubricates the joint) becomes inflamed. The inflammation eventually destroys the cartilage. As scar tissue gradually replaces the damaged cartilage, the joint becomes misshaped and rigid. Rheumatoid arthritis may damage the heart, lungs, nerves, eyes, and joints.

A medical examination and diagnosis is required to identify the cause and nature of any chronic joint or muscular pain. Other "rheumatic" diseases include arthralgia (pain in a joint), fibrositis ("muscular rheumatism"), and synovitis (inflammation of the joint membrane).

There is no simple cure for arthritis. Conventional treatment for chronic joint pain is to use drugs to suppress the inflammation in order to reduce pain and also prevent tissue destruction. Usually, simple aspirin-related pain medications, called nonsteroidal anti-inflammatory drugs (NSAIDs), are first prescribed. Corticosteroids may be prescribed for more serious illness, especially when tissue destruction is evident. In about fifteen percent of rheumatoid arthritis cases, these measures are ineffective, and stronger substances are used. Oral or injectable gold may prove helpful in treating rheumatoid arthritis. Some drugs usually used for cancer treatment may also be helpful.

Alternative physicians usually treat arthritis by recommending short fasts, screening for food allergies, recommending avoidance of processed foods, introducing fish and fish oils to the diet as well as anti-inflammatory herbal and nutritional supplements, and using natural methods to improve digestion. Alternative physicians may also recommend the substance glucosamine sulfate, which provides natural building blocks for cartilage, as a dietary supplement for those suffering from osteoarthritis. Scientific studies have suggested that supplementation with B vitamins, vitamin E, and some multiminerals (including the trace elements copper and selenium) may also improve the disease. On the other hand, studies have shown that nightshade vegetables—potatoes, tomatoes, bell peppers, and chili peppers—may provoke joint pain.

Very few of the herbs or foods recommended as a natural remedy for treating arthritis have been tested clinically for anti-inflammatory effects. Many of these herbs and foods contain plant constituents for which such effects are known, however.

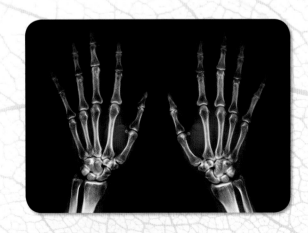

REMEDIES FOR ARTHRITIS

Celery

The remedy of eating raw or cooked celery seeds (*Apium graveolens*) or large amounts of the celery plant to treat rheumatism arrived in North America with the British and German immigrants. Using celery to treat rheumatism persists today in North American professional herbalism. Various parts of the celery plant contain more than twenty-five different anti-inflammatory compounds. And, taken as a food, celery is rich in minerals: A cup of celery contains more than 340 milligrams of potassium. (A potassium deficiency may contribute to some symptoms of arthritis.)

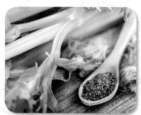

Directions: Place one teaspoon of celery seeds in a cup. Fill the cup with boiling water. Cover and let stand for fifteen minutes. Strain and drink three cups a day during an acute attacks.

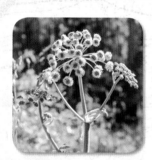

Angelica

Angelica (*Angelica archangelica*), an herb that has been used in European folk medicine since antiquity, can be used to treat arthritis. The Western variety of angelica has twelve anti-inflammatory constituents, ten antispasmodic (muscle relaxant) constituents, and five anodyne (pain-relieving) ones. The Chinese sometimes use their native variety of the plant (*Angelica sinensis*) for the same purpose. The Chinese species is sold in North America under the names *dang gui* or *dong quai*.

Directions: Place one tablespoon of the cut roots of either species of angelica in one pint of water and bring to a boil. Cover and boil for two minutes. Remove from heat and let stand, covered, until the water cools to room temperature. Strain and drink the tea in three doses during the day for two to three weeks at a time. Then, take a break for seven to ten days and start the treatment again if desired.

Rosemary

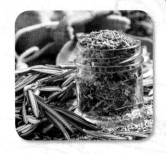

A collection of remedies by folklorist Clarence Meyer called *American Folk Medicine* suggests drinking rosemary tea to treat arthritis. The same remedy is used in the contemporary natural medicine of the Coahuila Indians in Mexico. Rosemary has not been tested in clinical trials, but it was used to relieve pain and spasm by doctors of the Physiomedicalist school, a group of M.D.s in the second half of the 19th century who used only herbs when treating patients. The plant's leaves contain four anti-inflammatory substances—carnosol, oleanolic acid, rosmarinic acid, and ursolic acid. Carnosol acts on the same anti-inflammatory pathways as both steroids and aspirin, oleanolic acid has been marketed as an antioxidant in China, rosmarinic acid acts as an anti-inflammatory, and ursolic acid, which makes up about four percent of the plant by weight, has been shown to have antiarthritic effects in animal trials.

Directions: Put ½ ounce of rosemary leaves in a one-quart canning jar and fill the jar with boiling water. Cover tightly and let stand for thirty minutes. Drink a cup of the hot tea before going to bed and have another cupful in the morning before breakfast. Do this for two to three weeks, and then take a break for seven to ten days before starting the treatment again.

Wintergreen

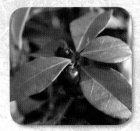

Wintergreen (*Gaulteria procumbens*) was used to treat arthritis by the Delaware, Menominee, Ojibwa, Potawatomi, and Iroquois Indian tribes. The plant was accepted in the United States as an official medicine for arthritis in 1820; it is still included—in the form of wintergreen oil—in the United States Pharmacopoeia today. The chief active pain-relieving constituent in wintergreen is methyl-salicylate. This compound can be toxic when consumed in concentrated wintergreen oil, even when applied to the skin, so, if you want to use this plant, stick with using the dried herb. (Aspirin was developed as a safer alternative to methyl-salicylate.)

Directions: Place one or two teaspoons of dried wintergreen leaves in a cup and cover with boiling water. Cover and let steep for fifteen minutes. Strain and drink three cups a day. Do this for two to three weeks, and then take a break for seven to ten days before starting again.

Arthritis

Black Cohosh

An American Indian treatment for arthritis, in both the Seneca and Cherokee tribes, involved using the root of black cohosh (*Cimicifuga racemosa*). White settlers in the eastern states eventually adopted the plant's use, as did the Eclectic physicians of the last century. There are five species in the *Cimicifuga* genus worldwide that have been used to treat rheumatism. Black cohosh contains aspirin-like substances as well as other anti-inflammatory and antispasmodic constituents.

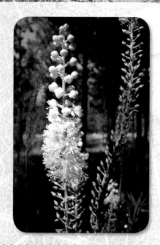

Directions: Simmer one teaspoon of black cohosh root in one cup of boiling water for twenty minutes. Strain and drink the tea in two divided doses during the day. Do this for two to three weeks. Take a break for seven to ten days before starting the treatment again.

Alfalfa

Alfalfa (*Medicago sativa*) is often promoted in health food stores as an arthritis remedy—in the form of capsulated alfalfa powder. Alfalfa contains L-canavanine, however, an amino acid that can cause symptoms that are similar to those of systemic lupus, an autoimmune disease that can also cause joint pain. Some scientific

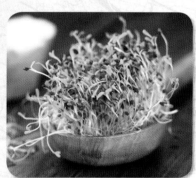

studies show that these symptoms can occur in both animals and humans as a result of eating alfalfa. Thus, the remedy below is best taken in the form of a tea rather than powder; the amino acid is not present to any significant amount in alfalfa tea. Alfalfa tea is rich with nutritive minerals. It is a recommended natural remedy for arthritis in southern Appalachia.

Directions: Place one ounce of alfalfa tea in a pot. Cover with one quart of water and boil for thirty minutes. Strain and drink the quart throughout the day. Do this for two to three weeks, and then take a break for seven to ten days before starting again.

Sesame Seeds

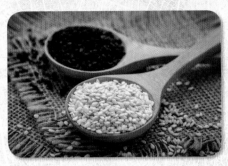

A remedy for arthritis from Chinese medicine is to eat sesame seeds. A half ounce of the seeds contains about 4 grams of essential fatty acids, 175 milligrams of calcium, 64 milligrams of magnesium, and, notably, .73 milligrams of copper. Increased copper intake may be important during arthritis attacks because the body's requirements go up during inflammation.

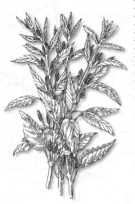

Directions: Grind up ½ ounce of sesame seeds in a coffee grinder and sprinkle on your food at mealtime. You can use this treatment for as long as you like.

Mustard Plaster

Perhaps the most famous of the counterirritant treatments for arthritis is the mustard plaster. This treatment is used throughout Europe and also in Appalachia and China. The irritating substance in mustard is allyl-isothyocyanate, which is related to the acrid substances in garlic and onions. This constituent is not activated, however, until the seeds are crushed and mixed with some liquid. Only then does the mustard produce the irritation necessary for the counterirritant effect.

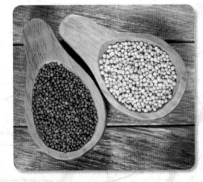

Directions: Crush the seeds of white or brown mustard (*Brassica alba, Brassica juncea*) or grind them in a seed grinder. Moisten the mixture with vinegar, then sprinkle with flour. Spread the mixture on a cloth. Place the cloth, poultice side down, on the skin. Leave on for no more than twenty minutes. Remove if the poultice becomes uncomfortable. After removing the poultice, wash the affected area.

Hot Peppers

Cayenne pepper (*Capsicum* spp.) appears in counterirritant potions in China, the American Southwest, and throughout Ohio, Indiana, and Illinois. External and internal use of cayenne pepper was a key element of Thomsonian herbalism, which was popular throughout rural New England and the Midwest in the early 1800s. Cayenne works by reduc-

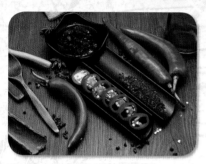

ing substance P, a chemical that carries pain messages from the skin's nerve endings, so it reduces pain when applied topically. Try this simple cayenne liniment.

Directions: Place one ounce of cayenne pepper in one quart of rubbing alcohol (a poison not for internal use). Let stand for three weeks, shaking the bottle each day. Then, using a cloth, apply to the affected area during acute attacks of pain. Leave the solution in place for ten to twenty minutes, then wipe clean.

Ginseng Liquor

The Iroquois Indians used American ginseng (*Panax quinquefolius*) as a treatment for rheumatism. Today, the Chinese use the herb for the same purpose. Be sure to use American ginseng, however, not Asian ginseng (*Panax ginseng*); Asian ginseng can actually aggravate the pain of arthritis. Ginseng contains constituents called ginsenosides, which have a variety of pharmacological actions. Both the American and Asian varieties of the plant are classified as adaptogens, meaning that they increase the body's ability to handle a wide variety of stresses. The Iroquois Indians made a tea of the plant's roots and added whiskey. You might prefer the traditional Chinese formula below.

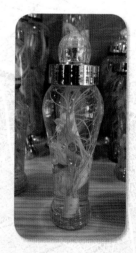

Directions: Chop three and a half ounces of ginseng and place in one quart of liquor like vodka. Let the mixture stand for five to six weeks in a cool dark place, turning the container frequently. Strain and take one ounce of the liquid after dinner or before bedtime every night for up to three months. Then, take a break for two weeks before starting the treatment again.

Hop Tea

Hop is native to Europe and can be found in vacant fields and along rivers there. The Pilgrims brought hop (*Humulus lupulus*) to Massachusetts, and it quickly spread south to Virginia. The hop plant contains at least twenty-two constituents that have anti-inflammatory activities, including

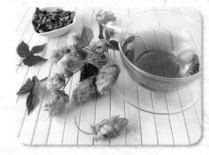

several that act through the same cellular mechanisms as steroid drugs. Four constituents have antispasmodic properties, and ten may act as sedatives. Today, a popular remedy for rheumatism in Mexico and the American Southwest is hop tea.

Directions: Place two or three teaspoons of hop leaves in a cup and fill with boiling water. Cover the cup and let stand for fifteen minutes. Drink the tea while it's warm. The tea is bitter. Drink one to three cups between dinner and bedtime as needed.

Wild Yam

Wild yam (*Dioscorea villosa*) was used by physicians of the last century to treat spasms of smooth muscle that often accompany gallbladder attacks or painful menstruation. Wild yam contains diosgenin, a steroid constituent with anti-inflammatory properties. Wild yam root itself has not been tested for such activity. Some southern African-Americans drink a tea of wild yam to treat muscular rheumatism. (Some eat the root of the wild yam instead.) This remedy was learned from the American Indians and is also recorded in the folk literature of contemporary whites in the Appalachian mountains of northern Georgia.

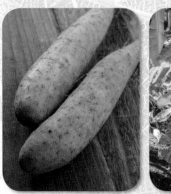
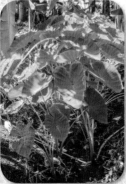

Directions: Place one ounce of wild yam root in a one-quart canning jar. Add a few slices of fresh ginger root. Fill the jar with boiling water, put the lid on tightly, and let the mixture stand until it reaches room temperature. Drink three cups each day for three, then take a break for seven to ten days.

Copper Bracelets

The recommendation for arthritis patients to wear copper bracelets is common throughout European and American folk literature. Copper is a nutrient that may play a role in modifying arthritis. The nutrient takes part in key antioxidant systems that help prevent inflammation and is also necessary for 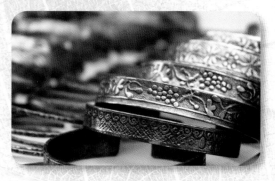 the formation of connective tissue. The normal daily requirement of copper for an adult is 1.5 to 3 milligrams, but that requirement may be higher in patients with rheumatoid arthritis (but not osteoarthritis). A 1976 clinical trial demonstrated that copper bracelets could be an effective treatment for arthritis. Patients in the trial who wore copper bracelets had fewer symptoms than those who wore colored aluminum look-alikes. The researchers also found that the bracelets lost as much as 1.7 milligrams of copper a day, some of which may have dissolved in the individual's sweat and been absorbed through the skin.

Directions: Wear a copper bracelet around your wrist or ankle—the more surface area the bracelet covers, the better. (It is unlikely to absorb too much copper. Copper toxicity occurs after ingesting about 60 milligrams of copper, an amount that is many times more than what is found in copper jewelry.)

Hydrotherapy

Water treatments for arthritis, which have become popular throughout the United States in the last century, invariably in- 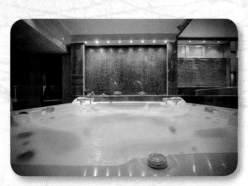 volve heat. Hot water or steam increases the circulation, which in turn can reduce local inflammation and swelling. These techniques are used today in parts of Appalachia and among the Seventh Day Adventists.

Directions: Try one of the following treatments: Take a steam bath in a sauna. Soak in a hot tub, or, if there is one in your area, a hot spring. You can also try placing hot towels on the afflicted area.

Epsom Salts

In the town of Epsom, England, in 1618, a substance called magnesium sulfate was found in abundance in spring water. The colonists brought the substance, named Epsom salts, to this country. Magnesium has both anti-inflammatory and antiarthritic properties and it can be absorbed through the skin. Magnesium is one of the most important of the essential minerals in the body, and it is commonly deficient in

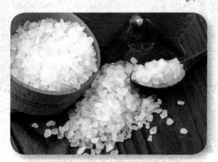

the American diet. A New England remedy for arthritis is a hot bath of Epsom salts. The heat of the bath can increase circulation and reduce the swelling and pain of arthritis.

Directions: Fill a bathtub with water as hot as you can stand. Add two cups of Epsom salts. Bathe for thirty minutes, adding hot water as necessary to keep the temperature warm. Do this daily as often as you'd like. (If you are pregnant or have cardiovascular disease, however, consult your doctor before taking very hot baths.)

Stinging Nettle

A Romani remedy for arthritis is to drink the juice of nettle leaves. Stinging nettle is an official remedy for rheumatism in Germany. In botanical medicine classes at the National College of Naturopathic Medicine in the United States, it is taught that stinging nettle is the most important herb to consider for treating early-onset arthritis. A 1996 laboratory analysis of nettle juice showed an anti-inflammatory effect similar to that of steroid drugs.

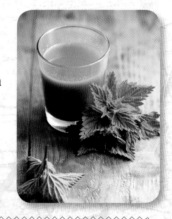

Directions: Purchase nettle leaf juice in a health food store and take as directed on the package. If you know how to identify and harvest nettles, collect your own (they must be harvested before they flower), and juice them in a juicer. Take one tablespoon of nettle juice three times a day. You can freeze the juice for later use. Also, you can make a tea of the dried leaves. Place one ounce of dried nettle in one quart of water. Bring to a boil and then simmer for thirty minutes. Drink three cups a day for as long as you'd like.

Arthritis

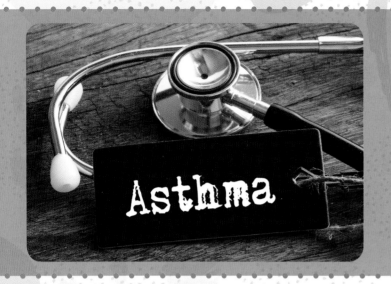

The suffocating symptoms of asthma are much more frequent in our society today than in the times of our ancestors. In fact, just since 1980, the incidence of asthma has risen more than sixty percent in the United States.

Asthma now affects some fourteen million Americans and claims about five thousand lives a year. Asthma is the most common chronic disease among children, affecting one in five. Because it may be a life-threatening condition, any individual with asthma should be under the care of a physician.

Asthma is a respiratory disorder marked by unpredictable periods of acute breathlessness and wheezing. Asthma attacks can last from less than an hour to a week or more and can strike frequently or only every few years. Attacks may be mild or severe and can occur at any time, even during sleep.

The difficult breathing occurs when the small respiratory tubes called bronchioles constrict or become clogged with mucus or when the membranes lining the bronchioles become swollen. When this happens, stale air cannot be fully exhaled but stays trapped in the lungs, so that less fresh air can be inhaled.

Asthma attacks can result from oversensitivity of the bronchial system to a variety of outside substances or conditions. About half of all asthma attacks are triggered by allergies to such substances as dust, smoke, pollen, feathers, pet hair, insects, mold spores, and a variety of foods and drugs. The al-

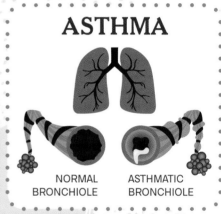

lergic trigger cannot always be identified, and sometimes food allergens complicate the picture. An individual who is allergic to a specific food may experience "allergic overload" when consuming it and then overreact to a simple pollen or other airborne allergen that normally would not cause a serious problem. Attacks not related to allergies can be set off by strenuous exercise,

44

breathing cold air, stress, and infections of the respiratory tract.

Modern physicians treat asthma with drugs delivered by inhalers, including, in serious cases, steroid drugs. Recent research has demonstrated that prolonged use of inhaled steroids can cause severe side effects similar to those experienced by users of oral steroids, however. Inhaled steroids nevertheless remain an essential and sometimes lifesaving part of treatment for severe asthma.

Why does the body overreact to a simple allergen? One possible explanation is a deficiency of the body's natural anti-inflammatory prostaglandins, substances naturally derived from the fats of cold water fish and wild game. The decline of these foods in the modern diet may be contributing to the increased incidence of asthma. The body can make these substances from certain vegetable oils, but the process is much more complex and can be inhibited by deficiencies of magnesium,

zinc, vitamin B6 or vitamin C—all common deficiencies in the modern American diet. Science has linked each of these deficiencies—as well as the reduced consumption of cold water fish—to asthma, but the evidence is not strong enough to implicate a single deficiency in all cases. Modern science has also demonstrated that increased salt consumption worsens (and reduced salt consumption improves) the severity of asthma. Although controversial, the industrialization of agriculture and food processing over the last few decades may have contributed to the increased incidence of asthma by exacerbating these deficiencies or excesses. Charles Cropley, a naturopathic physician in Colorado, recently described his dietary regimen for patients with asthma: "Nothing out of a can, nothing out of a box."

If you suffer from asthma, you might want to consider the natural remedies below. After

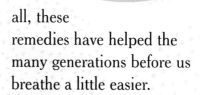

all, these remedies have helped the many generations before us breathe a little easier.

Amish Wisdom

The basic Amish treatment program for asthma includes eliminating all refined foods—such as sugar, flour, soft drinks, homogenized milk, coffee, black tea, and chocolate—from the diet. Prudent avoidance of airborne allergens is also a customary treatment of asthma among the Amish.

Asthma

Remedies for ASTHMA

Mormon Tea

Mormon tea, the common name for a variety of plants in the *Ephedra* genus, was used as a decongestant for allergies in western American natural medicine among American Indians, Hispanics, and settlers from the eastern states. A more potent Asian relative called *ma huang* is used in the same way in traditional Chinese medicine.

The medicinal constituents involved are ephedrine and pseudoephedrine, which also appear in over-the-counter allergy medicines. The American ephedra species do not contain reliable amounts of these constituents. *Ma huang* and ephedrine-containing drug combinations have been responsible for a number of deaths in the United States in recent years, but generally not when taken as allergy medications. Weight-loss formulas and pep pills sometimes contain *ma huang* or ephedrine. In this form they are consumed in much larger amounts than in allergy medications and present a greater risk of side effects. Ephedra is contraindicated in heart disease, hypertension, thyroid conditions, prostate disease, anxiety, pregnancy, and concurrent use of pharmaceutical drugs, except with approval of your physician. Mormon tea itself is not usually available in herb or health food stores, but *ma huang* often is.

DIRECTIONS: Cover one teaspoon of Chinese ephedra with one cup of boiling water. Let steep ten minutes. Drink the full cup when suffering an acute asthma attack. Prepare the tea ahead of time and keep it in a sealed container in the refrigerator.

46

Licorice

Licorice root has long been used to treat coughs and bronchial problems in many cultures throughout the world. It has expectorant properties and also contains anti-inflammatory constituents similar to steroids, although much weaker. Licorice is not so effective in treating an acute asthma attack, but daily use over a long period of time may reduce the body's tendency to overreact to allergens.

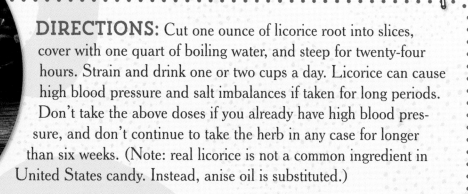

DIRECTIONS: Cut one ounce of licorice root into slices, cover with one quart of boiling water, and steep for twenty-four hours. Strain and drink one or two cups a day. Licorice can cause high blood pressure and salt imbalances if taken for long periods. Don't take the above doses if you already have high blood pressure, and don't continue to take the herb in any case for longer than six weeks. (Note: real licorice is not a common ingredient in United States candy. Instead, anise oil is substituted.)

Mustard Seed

An old New England remedy calls for one teaspoon of mustard seed (*Brassica* spp.), taken morning and evening, in the form of a tea or soup. Mustard contains irritating and expectorant sulfur-containing compounds. Like garlic, it can induce vomiting in larger doses and was used for this purpose by the Eclectic physicians of the late 19th and early 20th centuries in cases of narcotic poisoning.

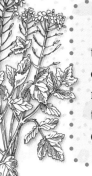

DIRECTIONS: Crush and moisten the seeds well in order to release the constituents. Let the freshly crushed mustard seeds sit in a warm soup or tea for ten to fifteen minutes before drinking. Take two to three times a day.

Garlic

Garlic (*Allium sativum*) has long been used to treat bronchial problems in many cultures. Like many of the other herbs used to treat asthma, garlic acts as an expectorant in low doses and an emetic in higher doses, especially if taken on an empty stomach. The Seventh Day Adventists use garlic in the following way to treat an acute asthma attack.

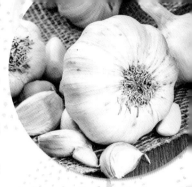

DIRECTIONS: Take two cloves of garlic and crush well or blend in a blender. Mix in two cups of hot water. Add a pinch of salt. Drink one cup rapidly. (Though this remedy may induce vomiting, it may also abort the asthma attack.) Then drink a second cup, which will usually stay down better than the first.

Also, you can try simmering the garlic in water for twenty minutes. (This destroys some of the irritating substances that cause nausea.) This treatment came from the 12th century German mystic Hildegarde von Bingen.

Honey

Honey has been used in traditional Chinese medicine for more than two thousand years. It is used to treat conditions ranging from asthma, cough, and chronic bronchitis to stomachache, constipation, chronic sinus congestion, canker sores, and burns. To cure a cough, a simple remedy from China recommends drinking a tea consisting of hot water and a tablespoon of honey. (This treatment probably isn't strong enough to treat an asthma attack, but it might help thin mucus and prevent congestion.) Expectorant syrups made from honey or sugar are widespread throughout the dolf traditions of the world. In the United States, honey syrups appear in the medicine of New England, Appalachia, and the Southwest.

Garlic & Honey

Some syrups combine the healthy benefits of both garlic and honey. Such syrups appear in the traditions of both New England and the Southwest.

DIRECTIONS: Place eight ounces of peeled and sliced garlic in one pint of boiling water. Let soak for ten to twelve hours, keeping the water warm, but not boiling. Strain and add two pounds of honey. Take one teaspoon of the mixture when you're congested.

Mullein & Honey

You can use the mullein plant to make an asthma syrup, too. Mullein (*Verbascum thapsus*) came from Europe to North America with the European colonists and is now naturalized throughout the United States and Canada. Its use as a cough medicine was quickly adopted by various Indian tribes, including the Mohegan, Delaware, Cherokee, Creek, and Navaho. The Penobscot, Potawatomi, and Iroquois used mullein specifically to treat asthma. It was an official medicine in the United States Pharmacopoeia from 1888 to 1936. Today, it is an approved medicine for treating coughs in Germany.

DIRECTIONS: Place ½ pound of mullein leaves in a one-quart jar. Fill the jar with boiling water and let cool to room temperature. Strain. Add honey to the tea until it is the consistency of syrup. Take one tablespoon of the syrup when suffering an asthma attack.

Nettle & Honey

This home remedy comes from German immigrants who settled in the New York area. Nettle juice (*Urtica dioica, Urtica urens*) and nettle syrups may still be purchased in Germany today. American physicians of the 19th and early 20th centuries also used nettle to treat some types of allergic conditions. Nettle is an unusually mineral-rich plant. An ounce of the dried herb contains more than two-thirds of the minimum daily requirement of magnesium, which is a frequently deficient mineral in asthma patients.

DIRECTIONS: Take ½ pint of nettle juice, boil it, remove the scum from the pot, and mix the remaining juice with an equal part of honey. Take one tablespoonful in the morning and evening.

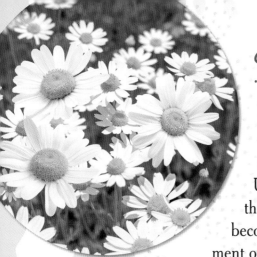

Daisy Blossoms

White daisy blossoms (*Chrysanthemum leucanthemum*) were an early traditional asthma remedy in the eastern United States. By the turn of the 20th century, this plant had become a standard medical treatment of the Eclectic physicians.

DIRECTIONS: Take four ounces of white daisy blossoms and crush them well. Pour one pint of boiling water over them. Steep for one hour and strain. Take three tablespoons two to three times a day.

Elder Flower Pillow

Another remedy from the eastern states of the last century is to sleep on a pillow stuffed with dried elder leaves or flowers (*Sambucus* spp.). As you sleep, you'll inhale the plant's aromatic oils and breathe a little easier.

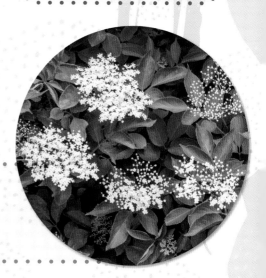

DIRECTIONS: Take four ounces of dried elder leaves or flowers and place inside a pillow. (Be careful of allergic reactions to the flower's pollen.)

Foot Bath & Tea

A Seventh Day Adventist treatment for asthma is to induce sweating by putting the feet in warm water and drinking a tea made of catnip (*Napeta cataria*) or pennyroyal (*Hedeoma pulegioides*). Catnip and pennyroyal are both diaphoretics—they bring circulation to the skin and produce sweating. Don't use this treatment during pregnancy, however; both these herbs promote menstruation.

DIRECTIONS: Fill a bathtub or a smaller tub with hot water. Put the feet in the water while drinking the hot tea. (This treatment is contraindicated in diabetics, however, because the feet might be burned.)

To make the tea, place one ounce of catnip or pennyroyal leaves in a one-quart jar and cover with boiling water. Cover the jar tightly and let steep for ten to fifteen minutes. Strain and drink.

Eggshells & Molasses

An early 18th century asthma treatment in the eastern United States was to mix roasted egg-shells with blackstrap molasses. This mixture makes an effective mineral supplement. The eggshells are almost pure calcium carbonate, and molasses is one of the most mineral-rich foods on earth. The dose of molasses below contains a significant portion of the recommended dietary allowance of magnesium, and this amount has been found in some scientific studies to be an effective treatment for asthma. (The treatment is remarkably similar to a traditional Mongolian remedy for leg cramps due to calcium deficiency, where black pepper berries are mixed with eggshells, which are roasted until brown and then crushed into powder.)

DIRECTIONS: Roast three eggshells until brown. Crush into a powder. Mix with half of a pint of molasses. The dose is one tablespoonful three times a day for as long as desired.

Herbal Formula

A tea formula from the last century combines licorice root (*Glycyrrhiza glabra*), mullein leaves (*Verbascum thapsus*), horehound leaves (*Marrubium vulgare*), lungwort (*Pulmonaria officinalis*), and sage (*Salvia officinalis*). All these herbs have subsequently been used in North American, British, and German herbal medicine, and licorice, mullein, horehound, and sage have all been listed as official medicines in the United States Pharmacopoeia.

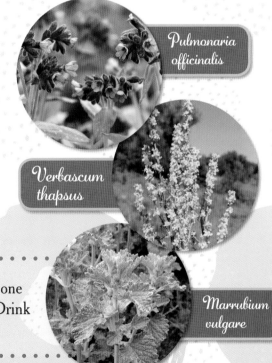

Pulmonaria officinalis

Verbascum thapsus

Marrubium vulgare

DIRECTIONS: Place ½ ounce of each of the herbs in one quart of water. Boil for twenty minutes. Strain when cool. Drink five ounces at bedtime.

Asthma

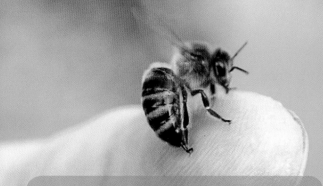

Humans, insects, and reptiles all strive to live comfortably in the same space. Unfortunately, humans inevitably get bitten and stung as a result.

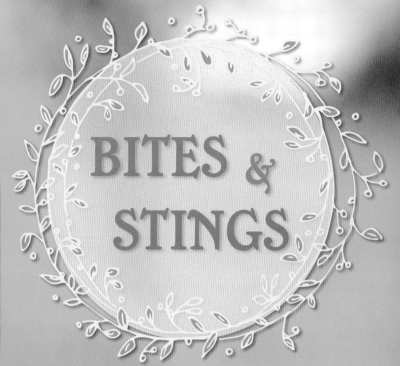

BITES & STINGS

When bees, wasps, scorpions, and snakes attack humans, it's usually because we threatened them or their living space. On the other hand, insects such as mosquitoes, biting flies, ticks, chiggers, and fleas are predatory pests that view humans as good opportunities for a bite to eat. Their bites are more likely to be itchy than painful. With any bite or sting, the species' venom, or sometimes the tiny insect itself penetrates the barriers of the body. The combination of the effects of the poison and the body's attempt to eliminate it can cause pain, swelling, or itching near the bite site.

Most bites and stings are not a serious medical concern, but there are a few exceptions. In some people, the stings of bees, wasps, and hornets can cause a potentially fatal allergic reaction called anaphylactic shock. Any shortness of breath, difficulty breathing, or swelling in the airway after a sting is a medical emergency requiring immediate attention. Tick bites can cause Lyme disease or Rocky Mountain spotted fever. Bites of the black widow spider and brown recluse spider can also cause serious medical symptoms; any reaction following a spider bite requires medical attention.

The bites of the poisonous snakes in North America are not usually life threatening to healthy adults. Of about eight thousand such bites

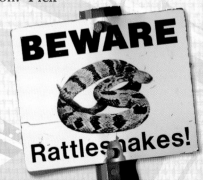

BEWARE Rattlesnakes!

in the United States each year, fewer than fifteen cause fatalities; the deaths occur mostly in children and the elderly. The illness from a poisonous snake bite can be quite severe, however, and should be treated as a medical emergency. Any snake bite can cause an infected puncture wound, which requires careful cleaning and medical attention.

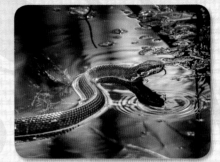

The *Centruroides exilicauda* scorpion, native to Arizona, New Mexico, and the California side of the Colorado River, is the only North American scorpion that can cause serious illness or death. The folk remedies here are for normal itches and pains associated with bites and stings, not for the more exotic complications caused by Lyme disease, anaphylactic shock, or snake bites.

My Scorpion Bite

Once in Arizona, I was bitten by a *Centruroides exilicauda* scorpion, the only potentially lethal poisonous scorpion in North America. I didn't know I'd been bitten, but thought I'd been stabbed by a cactus thorn. Soon my arm was numb, an itchy rash crept under my legs to the knees, and my pulse rate rose to more than 100 beats per minute. I went to bed but didn't figure what had happened until I woke the next morning and my heart rate was still over 100 beats per minute. I soon realized it was a scorpion bite and took the Plain

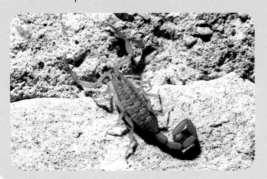

Indians' remedy for rattlesnake bites, *Enchinacea angustifoli*. Nothing happened at first, but within five hours I fell asleep and woke up as if nothing happened. I was left with a small scar and an appreciation for natural remedies. —P. Bergner

53

Remedies for
BITES & STINGS

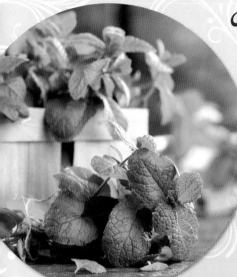

Mints

American Indian tribes have used various species of mint for the relief and prevention of insect bites. For example, peppermint (*Mentha piperita*) contains camphor, which is cooling to the skin and helps to relieve itching.

Directions: Place one ounce of peppermint leaf in a one-quart canning jar and cover with boiling water. Seal the jar and let stand until the water cools to room temperature. Apply to mosquito bites or other itchy areas with a cloth. Reapply as desired.

Pennyroyal

Early American colonists introduced European pennyroyal to North America, but found the Indians were already using American pennyroyal (*Hedeoma pulegioides*). The herb was used by American Indians to prevent deer tick bites. In the Frank C. Brown *Collection of North Carolina Folklore*, a North Carolina source says: "Pennyroyal beaten on the legs will keep insects away." Pennyroyal contains eleven separate constituents with identified insect-repellent properties.

Directions: Purchase the essential oil of pennyroyal. Put eight to ten drops in some almond oil, mix, and apply—especially around the ankles, neck, and scalp—to repel ticks and other insects.

Tobacco

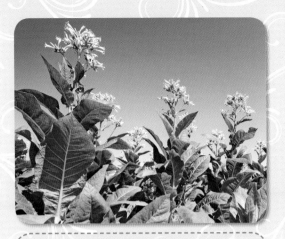

The Mayan Indians moistened the leaves of wild tobacco (*Nicotiana rustica, N. glauca*) with saliva and applied the leaves to a bite or sting. The Six Nations, a league of Indians that extended from the Hudson River to Lake Erie, also used tobacco to treat insect bites. Using tobacco in this manner later passed into Appalachian folk medicine, where tobacco poultices are still used today to treat bee, hornet, yellow jacket, and wasp stings as well as spider bites. In the folk medicine of the Southwest, a strong tobacco tea is applied to tick bites to help draw the tick out. Physicians of the last century also supported tobacco's antiseptic qualities: They used tobacco ointments and tobacco poultices to treat skin conditions.

Directions: Mix tobacco from cigarettes, cigars, chewing tobacco, or snuff with water and apply directly to a bite or sting. Leave the mixture on as long as you like.

Echinacea

Echinacea (*Echinacea angustifolia, E. purpurea*), also known as Kansas snakeroot, was a snakebite remedy of the Plains Indians introduced into medical practice in the United States in the mid-1880s. Dr. H.F.C. Meyer, M.D., a Nebraska doctor, learned how to use echinacea to treat snakebites from an American Indian woman. He experimented with the plant for about fifteen years; he even injected himself with rattlesnake poison and used the plant as an antidote. Echinacea was later identified by science as an immune stimulant. Today, it is one of the most popular herbal remedies in North America and in Europe, especially in Germany, where it is prescribed by physicians for colds, flu, and infections.

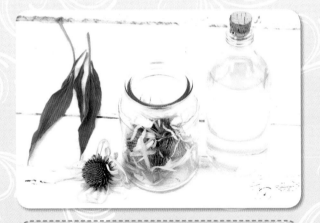

Directions: Take a tincture of echinacea root with you when hiking in rattlesnake country. If bitten by a snake, take a one-teaspoon dose every half an hour and drink plenty of liquids. Snakebites are considered a medical emergency, however, so you should go to a medical facility as soon as possible.

Bites & Stings

Plantain Leaves

Plantain (*Plantago* spp.), the common four-leafed weed that grows in lawns and around sidewalks throughout the country, was once called "White Man's Footprint" by the eastern American Indians because it came to this country with the European immigrants and spread wherever they went. Various tribes quickly adopted the plant as a medicine for treating bites, stings, and minor wounds. The Six Nations used the plant specifically to treat spider bites. Plantain leaves are still used today in the natural medicine of Indiana, North Carolina, and the Southwest. Plantain's chemical constituents may explain its ability to soothe pain and promote wound healing: It contains at least fifteen constituents with identified anti-inflammatory properties, seventeen with bactericidal properties, six analgesics, and five antiseptics. It also contains the constituent allantoin, which promotes cell proliferation and tissue healing.

Directions: Crush a small handful of fresh plantain leaves and apply locally to bites and stings. Applied externally, the plant stimulates and cleanses the skin and encourages wounds to heal faster. You can apply fresh leaves every fifteen to twenty minutes. Leave on as long as desired.

Vinegar

In the folklore of New England, rural Indiana, the American Southwest, and among the Romani and the Amish, a vinegar wash is recommended for treating bites and stings.

Directions: Use undiluted vinegar as a wash to stop itching or to relieve the pain of stings. Also, you can try this Romani recipe: Take a handful of thyme (*Thymus vulgaris*) and seal it in a bottle of vinegar for one cycle of the moon, in the sun if possible. Shake the bottle every morning and evening. Then, after an additional half cycle of the moon, crush seven garlic cloves and add them to the bottle. At the end of the second lunar cycle, strain and bottle the liquid. Use as a wash for itchy or infected bites.

Charcoal

A charcoal poultice is a medical treatment of the Seventh Day Adventists for insect and snake bites. Charcoal has strong drawing properties and is sometimes taken internally to neutralize ingested poisons in the gut.

Directions: Wet as much crushed charcoal as you need to cover the injured area. Place the charcoal directly over the area and cover with a clean cloth. Replace the poultice every ten to fifteen minutes until relief is obtained.

Clay

Using clay or mudpacks to treat bee and wasp stings seems to be a universal folk remedy. In North America, it appears in the folk literature of southern blacks, Canadians, New Englanders, New Yorkers, North Carolinians, the Aztec Indians of Mexico, and contemporary Hispanics in Texas and New Mexico. Some people believe it works by literally drawing the toxins out.

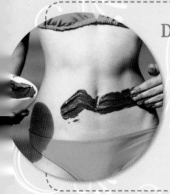

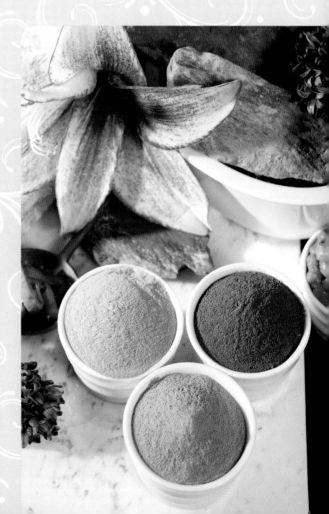

Directions: Apply mud or cold clay (any kind of clay soil or cosmetic clay will do) to the sting area to relieve pain and reduce swelling. When the clay dries, apply new clay. Repeat this as long as necessary.

57

BLADDER & KIDNEY

Be aware that changes in urine and urinary habits that do not seem to have an obvious cause may be a sign of disease.

The urinary system includes those organs of the body that produce or eliminate urine. By controlling urine flow, the system maintains proper water balance in the body. Changes in urine and urinary habits that do not seem to have an obvious cause may be symptoms of disease. An accurate diagnosis by a physician is the first step to proper treatment.

Most pathological conditions of the kidney and bladder are not appropriate for self-treatment with natural or home remedies. Even bladder infections, the least serious of common urinary tract conditions, require a diagnosis to rule out sexually transmit-ted diseases or more serious kidney involvement. Most of the natural remedies below for treating urinary tract infections work in the same way as conventional treatment recommendations, however. For example, drinking adequate water to wash out bacteria is a standard procedure in both folk and conventional medicine for treating urinary tract infections.

Most of the natural remedies in this section use herbs with mild diuretic properties. These herbs increase the flow of urine through the urinary tract, helping to wash out irritating substances. In Germany, the use of such mild diuretics is called "flushing out therapy"; in that country, the therapy is a routine conventional treatment for bladder infections and stone prevention. Research has shown that mild diuretics increase urination and reduce joint swelling. Thus, mild natural diuretics are also used in Germany for treating the swollen joints of arthritis.

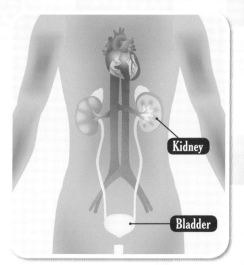

Kidney

Bladder

An important restriction on the use of herbal diuretics, however, is in cases of edema resulting from heart, kidney, or liver disease. (The condition was once known as "dropsy.") Edema requires careful medical attention—and properly monitored doses of diuretics. Although some natural remedies were once used to treat edema, during the 20th century, modern medical science has discovered much safer and more effective treatments for the condition.

The remedies in this section are found in many cultures throughout the world. In fact, most of these remedies would be included in classes on urinary tract herbs in medical schools in Germany, where doctors and pharmacists are required by law to receive training in medical herbalism.

A topic not included in this section is urinary difficulties due to prostate problems. Any obstructive problems of the urinary tract due to enlargement of the prostate require conventional medical attention to determine the cause.

Kidney Stones

A myth perpetuated in many modern herbals and collections of natural remedies is that certain herbs or foods will "dissolve stones." Kidney stones are formed when certain salts become too concentrated in the urine. Once formed, they do not readily dissolve back into the urine, however, and must either pass down the urinary tract or be broken up or dissolved by conventional medical means. Certain individuals, sometimes referred to in conventional medicine as "stone formers," tend to suffer repeat attacks of kidney stones. For them, the best treatment for kidney stones is prevention, which involves drinking plenty of water to dilute the urine. Drinking large amounts of fluids, particularly at night, reduces urine concentration so that stones cannot form.

kidney stones

Remedies for
BLADDER & KIDNEY ISSUES

Bearberry

The herb bearberry (*Arctostaphylos uva ursi*), sometimes called *uva ursi* (bearberry in Latin), was first recorded as a medicinal herb in the 13th century Welsh herbal book *The Physicians of Myddfai*. The berries of the plant are a favorite food of bears—thus its name. Its use as a diuretic and lower urinary tract disinfectant is recorded in subsequent centuries throughout the British Isles and northern Europe. American Indians, including the Cheyenne and Thompson tribes, have used the plant for the same purposes. Today, bearberry is used as a diuretic in the medicine of Indiana and also by Spanish Gypsies from Spain.

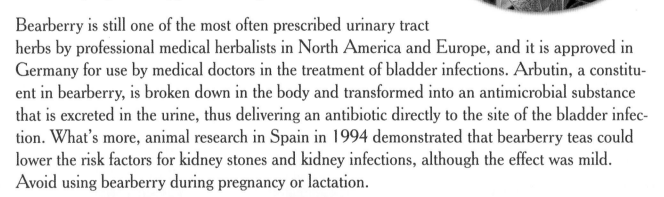

Bearberry is still one of the most often prescribed urinary tract herbs by professional medical herbalists in North America and Europe, and it is approved in Germany for use by medical doctors in the treatment of bladder infections. Arbutin, a constituent in bearberry, is broken down in the body and transformed into an antimicrobial substance that is excreted in the urine, thus delivering an antibiotic directly to the site of the bladder infection. What's more, animal research in Spain in 1994 demonstrated that bearberry teas could lower the risk factors for kidney stones and kidney infections, although the effect was mild. Avoid using bearberry during pregnancy or lactation.

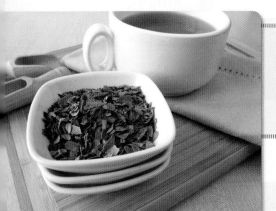

Directions: Simmer ½ ounce of bearberry leaves in one pint of water for five minutes. Let steep until the water reaches room temperature. For a bladder infection, strain and drink one ounce three times a day for up to five days.

Corn Silk

Corn silk (*Zea mays*), the hairy projections from the end of an ear of corn, was introduced as a medicine to the Western world after the European conquest of Mexico, Central America, and South America. Corn, native to those areas, is now cultivated not only in the Americas, but as far away as Africa, India, and China. Corn silk tea was used as a diuretic by American Indians in the conquered regions and is now used in the same way in traditions throughout North America and Europe. It has even entered into formal Chinese medical traditions, where it is called *yu mi shu*. It is often prescribed as a diuretic by professional medical herbalists of Europe, North America, and Australia.

Directions: Fill a one-quart jar $\frac{1}{3}$ full of fresh corn silk. Pour enough boiling water to fill the jar, cover, and let cool to room temperature. Strain and drink the quart in four doses during the day for seven to ten days.

Goldenrod

If you're not allergic to this common cause of hay fever, goldenrod (*Solidago* spp.) may be as useful to you as a mild diuretic that helps to flush out the urinary tract. It was used for this purpose by the Chippewa Indians; it is used in the same way today in the natural medicine of Indiana. (Goldenrod was also used in Europe as a treatment for wounds—the flowers would be packed into a wound to stop the bleeding.) Goldenrod is approved for medical use in Germany as a mild diuretic and treatment for bladder infections.

Directions: Place a handful of goldenrod flowers in a one-pint jar and fill with boiling water. Cover and let cool to room temperature. To treat a bladder infection, strain and drink the pint in three doses during the day for seven to ten days.

Bladder & Kidney

"Joe-Pye" Weed

Queen of the meadow (*Eupatorium purpureum, Eupatorium maculatum*) was used medicinally by eastern American Indians, including the Cherokee and Mohawk tribes, before the arrival of European colonists. An Indian healer named Joe Pye reportedly used it to treat a group of colonists suffering from typhoid fever, and the survivors of the epidemic named the plant in honor of him—thus, Joe-Pye weed. It is also called "gravel root" because of its prominent use as a treatment for kidney stones. Queen of the meadow was used by Eclectic physicians from about 1848 until the group's demise in the 1940s. The Eclectics preferred Queen of the meadow over some other diuretic plants because of its mild, non-irritating effects. One of the Eclectic physicians, Harvey Felter, M.D., stated in a turn-of-the-century medical book, *King's American Dispensatory*, that the herb was effective in treating kidney stones for two reasons—first, because it increased the flow of urine, preventing stone formation or washing out existing stones, and second, it reduced inflammation and pain in the urinary tract. Felter disputed the common myth that the plant could dissolve kidney stones that had already formed, however.

Queen of the meadow is recommended in the remedies of North Carolina residents for treating or preventing painful urinary tract conditions. The plant is still prescribed as a diuretic for bladder infections and kidney stones by professional medical herbalists in North America, although it has not been used in North American or European conventional medicine since the time of the Eclectics.

Directions: Add ½ ounce of Queen of the meadow to a pint of water. (Queen of the meadow may be sold in your herb shop under the name "gravel root.") Cover and simmer for twenty minutes. Let cool to room temperature. Drink two to three cups a day, while also drinking plenty of water.

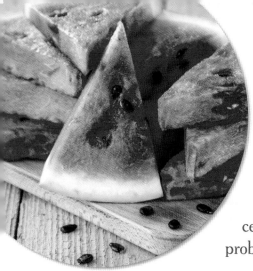

Watermelon

Watermelon seed tea (*Citrullus vulgaris*) is a natural diuretic mentioned in the literature of Indiana and North Carolina. It is also recommended by the Amish and the Seventh Day Adventists, the latter being a religious movement that advocates natural remedies and alternative medicine. Watermelon seed was also used as a diuretic by Eclectic physicians during the last century. Today, it is not commonly found in medical herbalism, probably because it is not always available in herb stores.

Directions: Place a handful of fresh watermelon seeds in the bottom of a one-pint jar and fill with boiling water. Let cool to room temperature. Strain and drink a pint of the tea each day for seven to ten days.

Pumpkin Seeds

Another diuretic often mentioned in natural remedy literature is pumpkin seeds (*Cucurbita pepo*). The medical traditions of New England, Indiana, and Louisiana all suggest taking a few pumpkin seeds to promote urination. The Eclectic physicians of the last century followed the practice until the group's demise in the 1940s.

Contemporary German physicians use pumpkin seed preparations to treat difficult urination that accompanies enlarged prostate (when prostate cancer as a cause has been ruled out). Two constituents in pumpkin seeds, adenosine and cucurbitacin, both have diuretic properties.

Directions: Crush a handful of fresh pumpkin seeds and place in the bottom of a one-pint jar. Fill with boiling water. Let cool to room temperature. Strain and drink a pint of the tea each day.

Also, you can eat pumpkin seeds according to taste. It is best to remove the shells and eat them with little or no salt.

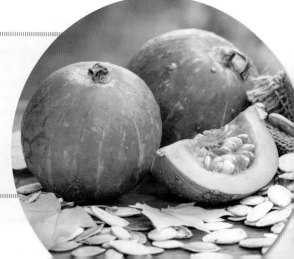

Juniper Berries

The ancient Egyptians used juniper berries as a diuretic. Juniper berries have been used for the same purpose by American Indians of the Tewa, Paiute, Shoshone, Cree-Hudson Bay, and Iroquois tribes. Today, juniper berries are recommended as a diuretic in the natural medicine of New England and the southern Appalachians. Contemporary medical herbalists warn that the aromatic oils in juniper berries can increase kidney irritation, and that it should not be used if kidney infection accompanies bladder infection. (The studies showing the resulting kidney irritation used concentrated oils in animals, not berries in humans, but due caution is in order.) Juniper berries are approved for use as a diuretic in Germany.

Cranberry Juice

One of the most famous natural remedies for bladder infections—widely followed today throughout North America—is to drink cranberry juice. This remedy is especially well known in the natural medicine of New England.

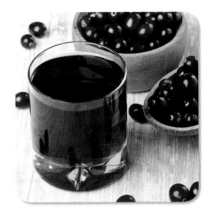

This remedy, which has been studied in modern clinical trials, has been found to be effective in preventing, but not treating, bladder infections. A study conducted at the Brigham and Women's Hospital in Boston, and published in the prestigious *Journal of the American Medical Association* in 1994, found that consumption of about twelve ounces of commercial cranberry juice each day for a month reduced bacterial counts in the lower urinary tracts of elderly women. Several other trials have shown similar results. (Using cranberry juice as a preventive may be very useful to bedridden elders, who are at higher risk for bladder infections.)

Constituents in the cranberry juice help to prevent bacteria from sticking to the walls of the urinary tract, making the bacteria easier to flush out. Once the infection is underway, however, and the bacteria have set up shop, the cranberry juice is not of much use.

Directions: Obtain a sugar-free cranberry juice or juice concentrate from a health food store. (The brands in supermarkets contain enough sugar to depress the activity of the immune system.) Drink eight to twelve ounces of the juice a day to prevent infections.

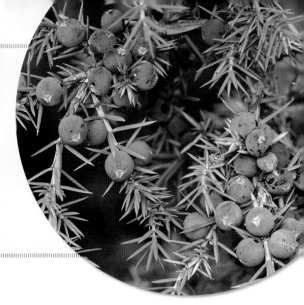

Directions: Place two tablespoons of juniper berries in the bottom of a one-pint jar. Fill with boiling water and cover tightly to prevent the escape of aromatic oils. Strain and drink the pint during the day. Do not try this remedy if you have kidney disease. The tea should not be consumed for more than three weeks. Take a break for two to three weeks between courses of treatment. This remedy should not be used by persons who have an existing renal disease.

Plants Containing Berberine

A New England remedy suggests using the plant goldthread (*Coptis trifolia*) to treat urinary tract infections. Drs. Agatha Thrash, M.D., and Calvin Thrash, M.D., authors in the tradition of the Seventh Day Adventists, suggest using goldenseal (*Hydrastis canadensis*) for the same purpose. Nineteenth-century physicians of the homeopathic school of medicine used tinctures of Oregon grape root (*Mahonia aquifolium, Berberis aquifolium*) for urinary tract infections.

Goldenseal

The three plants have a constituent in common, called berberine. Berberine has strong antibacterial properties. Berberine is not very well absorbed across the intestinal wall, though the most prominent use of these plants is for intestinal infections. The small amounts that are absorbed, however, are excreted through the kidneys and concentrated in the urine. This could explain the therapeutic effect, if any, on urinary tract infections. Goldthread is usually not available in the herb marketplace, and goldenseal is now an endangered species, facing extinction in North America. Oregon grape root is readily available at low cost, however.

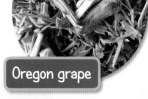

Oregon grape

Directions: To treat urinary tract infections, simmer one tablespoon of Oregon grape root in a pint of water for twenty minutes. Cool to room temperature. Strain and drink the pint during the day for seven to ten days.

Bladder & Kidney

Parsley

The ancient Egyptians, Greeks, and Romans all used parsley (*Petroselinum crispum*) as a diuretic. The practice continues today both by the Romani and in the tradition of New England. Parsley, which originated in the eastern Mediterranean region, was introduced to England in the year 1548, and within a hundred years, it was recommended in British medical herbals for use as a diuretic in cases of severe edema (dropsy).

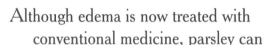

Although edema is now treated with conventional medicine, parsley can still be used to remedy other conditions. Parsley is approved by the German government for use as a mild diuretic and for treatment of bladder infections. For safety's sake, use parsley root rather than parsley seeds, parsley juice, or parsley leaves. (Parsley seeds can stimulate uterine contractions or irritate the kidneys. Parsley juice can also stimulate uterine contractions and should thus be avoided during pregnancy. And, although parsley leaves are nutritious, they do not contain much of the diuretic constituents of the plant.) The following formula is a modification of a Romani diuretic formula used for urinary tract infections and kidney stones.

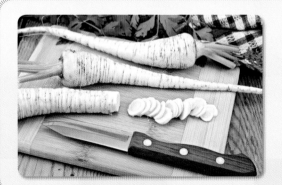

Directions: Take a handful of parsley roots and cut them into small pieces. Place them in one quart of water, bring to a boil, and simmer for ten to fifteen minutes. Remove from the heat and stir in a handful of rose blossoms. Steep, covered, for ten minutes. Strain and drink five to seven cups of the tea during the course of a day for seven to ten days. Do not use during pregnancy and lactation.

Anise

The Amish use anise seed (*Pimpinella anisum*) as a diuretic. Hispanics in the Southwest use it the same way—as did the ancient Egyptians and Greeks. The Greek herbalist Dioscorides, whose book of herbal medicine was used by doctors in Europe for at least 1600 years, stated that anise seed "provokes urine." Anise, better known in medical herbalism as a digestive stimulant, is probably one of the mildest diuretics in this section.

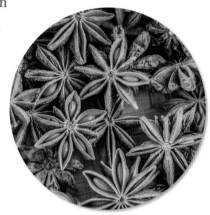

Directions: Crush one teaspoon of anise seeds in a grinder or with a mortar and pestle. Place in a cup and fill with boiling water. Cover well, and let steep for ten minutes. Strain and drink two to three cups a day. Don't take anise except as a simple food spice in pregnancy, because anise can stimulate uterine contractions when taking above dose.

Burdock

Burdock (*Arctium* spp.) has been used since ancient times as a mild diuretic. The Iroquois Indians used the root for this purpose. In 17th century Great Britain, the plant's seeds were used specifically for treating the bladder and kidney stones.

In Germany, burdock is commonly used in contemporary medical practice, even though a review by the German government failed to find adequate clinical research to justify its use. However, in 1994, animal research in Spain demonstrated that, while burdock root teas did lower the risk factors for kidney stones and kidney infections, the effect was mild. And, although burdock is widely used in contemporary North American professional herbalism, its most common use in this country is as a "blood cleanser," not as an effective diuretic.

Directions: Place one ounce of burdock root in one quart of water in a pot and simmer, covered, for twenty minutes. Let cool, strain, and drink the quart of tea throughout the day. Continue treatment for up to three weeks.

Bladder & Kidney

Water

The most obvious diuretic to increase the flow of urine is water. Simply drinking plenty of water—six to eight glasses a day—can increase urine flow, dilute the urine to prevent stone formation, and wash out bacteria that may cause infections. Some of the benefits of the mild diuretic teas used by physicians in Germany and by professional herbalists in North America come from the tea's increased volume of water. German physician R.F. Weiss, M.D., suggested that individuals who are prone to forming stones should, one day a week, consume a quart and a half of water rapidly (within fifteen minutes) to wash out any tiny stones that may be forming.

> **Directions:** Drink eight glasses of water a day. Or, one day a week, drink eight glasses of water in succession, within fifteen minutes, to flush out the urinary tract.

Horsetail

Horsetail (*Equisetum arvense*) was used as a medicine by the ancient Greeks. It has been used specifically as a diuretic in Western traditional medicine since the 1500s. The Iroquois Indians used a North American species of the plant (*Equisetum hymenale*) for the same purpose. Today, horsetail is used as a diuretic in the Hispanic natural medicine of the Southwest.

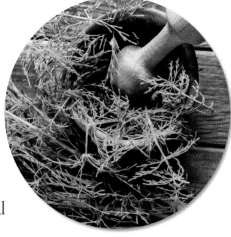

> **Directions:** Place one tablespoon of horsetail herb in a one-pint jar and cover with boiling water. Cover and let stand for ten to fifteen minutes. Strain and drink the pint in three doses throughout the day. Do not take horsetail for longer than three weeks on a daily basis; it can irritate the digestive tract when taken for long periods.

Horsetail is approved by the German government for use as a diuretic and for treatment of bladder infections. In 1994, animal research in Spain demonstrated that horsetail teas also lowered the risk factors for kidney stones and kidney infections, although the effect was mild. Note: Do not confuse this plant with marsh horsetail (*Equisetum palustre*), a larger plant that contains toxic alkaloids.

Buchu

The Hottentot tribe of southern Africa first acquainted Europeans with the use of buchu (*Barosma betulina*). In 1821, it was imported to England. By 1840, it appeared in the United States Pharmacopoeia as an official medicine; it remained listed in following editions until 1940. It was used for treating urinary tract infections by all schools of medicine during that period. (The Eclectic physicians cautioned that the plant's oils could further irritate those urinary tract infections that are accompanied by burning or stinging pain, however.) The plant's constituents are probably its aromatic peppermint-like oils. Buchu is used by conventional doctors in Germany as a mild diuretic and for treatment of bladder infections.

Buchu

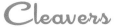

Marshmallow

Directions: Place ½ ounce of buchu leaves and ½ ounce of marshmallow root (*Althea officinalis*) in one quart of water. Cover the pot and simmer on the lowest heat for thirty to forty minutes. Allow to cool to room temperature. Strain and drink one-ounce doses three to four times a day for seven to ten days.

Cleavers

Cleavers (*Galium aparine*) is most commonly used in contemporary medical herbalism as a "blood cleanser" for skin conditions. But a tea made of cleavers—also known as goose grass or bed straw (it was also used to stuff mattresses)—has been used as a diuretic as well. The Ojibwa Indians used it for this purpose, as did the physicians of the Physiomedicalist and Eclectic schools—groups of doctors from the 19th and early 20th centuries who primarily used herbs as medicines.

Directions: Place one ounce of cleavers in a quart of water and simmer for ten to fifteen minutes. Let cool to room temperature. Drink the quart of tea in three to four divided doses through the day.

Bladder & Kidney

BOILS & CARBUNCLES

Boils can occur on any part of the body that has hair follicles. Thus, only the lips, palms, and soles of the feet can be spared.

Boils—furuncles is the medical term—are tender, inflamed swellings centered around hair follicles in the scalp or skin. They result from infection by various strains of *Staphylococcus* bacteria. Carbuncles are clusters of boils, often appearing on the nape of the neck. Boils and carbuncles may appear on otherwise healthy individuals, although diabetes mellitus, debilitating diseases, and old age may predispose a person to the condition. Boils do not normally present a health hazard, but carbuncles may be accompanied by fever and exhaustion. Boils on the nose or in the central area of the face require prompt medical attention and treatment with antibiotics, however, because the bacterial infection can spread easily from that area to the brain.

Conventional and traditional treatment for simple boils is identical: Applications of moist heat until the boil comes to a head and drains spontaneously. Surgical incision or squeezing can spread the infection internally and should be avoided. For more serious or recurrent infections, the conventional treatment is antibiotic therapy. Besides the use of poultices and disinfectant washes, traditional medicine and natural remedies also center on purifying the blood through building up the strength of the immune system to resist bacterial infection.

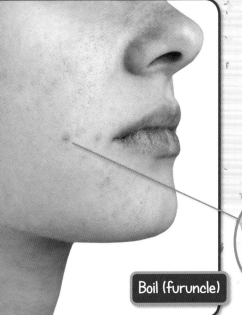

Boil (furuncle)

Remedies for BOILS & CARBUNCLES

Chamomile Poultice

The medicine of the American Southwest recommends a poultice of hot chamomile tea (*Matricaria recutita*) for treating boils. Chamomile contains essential oils that have antiseptic, antibacterial, and anti-inflammatory properties.

DIRECTIONS: Place ½ ounce of chamomile flowers in a one-pint canning jar and cover with boiling water. Cover the jar tightly and let stand for fifteen minutes. Strain the liquid and apply the hot mash directly to the boil. Cover with a cloth, and keep the cloth moist with the strained liquid. Do this remedy every two to three hours for twenty minutes at a time, until the boil comes to a head and drains.

Slippery Elm Poultice

An Appalachian remedy for boils combines hot water with slippery elm to make a paste. When mixed with water, shredded or powdered slippery elm bark (*Ulmus fulva*) makes a thick, sticky mass that can easily be applied to the skin. The mucilage in the bark soothes the tissues and the heat from the hot water draws blood to the area.

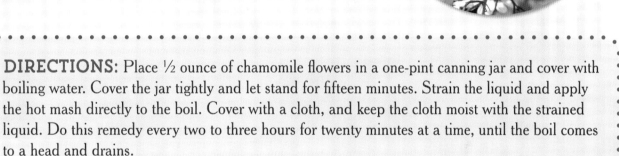

Slippery Elm

DIRECTIONS: In a pot, bring ½ cup of water to a boil. Turn off the heat and, stirring, add enough slippery elm bark powder to make a thick paste. Apply the paste directly to the boil, and cover with a cloth. Repeat every one to two hours until the boil comes to a head and drains spontaneously.

71

Cornmeal Poultice

A remedy of the Aztecs—which survives today in the medicine of the American Southwest—was to apply a poultice of cornmeal and hot water to the boil. The same method was used by the Cherokee Indians, who passed the remedy along to the Appalachians. The remedy is still used today in rural Indiana. It is the texture of the corn and its ability to hold the heat of water—not the medicinal properties of the corn—that are responsible for the value of this treatment.

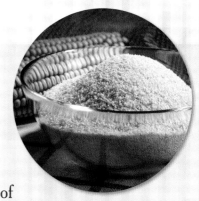

DIRECTIONS: In a pot, bring ½ cup of water to a boil. Turn off the heat and add cornmeal to make a thick paste. Apply the mixture to the boil, and cover with a cloth. Repeat every one to two hours until the boil comes to a head and drains.

Onion Poultice

Onion (*Allium cepa*) poultices were used among eastern American Indian tribes, European colonists of the eastern states, Appalachian healers, contemporary Indiana farmers, and contemporary Hispanic New Mexicans to treat boils. Onions contain antiseptic chemicals and irritating constituents that draw blood and heat to the affected area.

DIRECTIONS: Place a thick slice of onion over the boil and keep in place by wrapping with a cloth. Change every three to four hours until the boil comes to a head and drains.

Egg Skin Poultice

A 19th-century remedy for treating boils in the eastern United States was to apply the soft outer skin of a hard-boiled egg directly to the boil. It is now a commonly used remedy in contemporary New England, Appalachia, and southwestern Colorado.

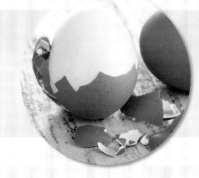

Flax Seeds & Oil

Poultices made of flax seeds or flax oil are recommended in the folk literature of New England, Appalachia, and Indiana. If flax-seed (linseed) oil is used instead of the seeds, it must be mixed with flour or cornmeal. Although flax seeds and flax oil are sometimes used medicinally for their essential fatty acid content to prevent inflammatory diseases, this probably has no local effect when applied topically. Any effect probably comes from the texture of the poultices rather than their constituents.

DIRECTIONS:
Grind one tablespoon of flax seeds. Add the seeds to ¼ cup of boiling water. Let the mixture become gelatinous. Cover the boil with a cloth, and then spread the flaxseed mush over it, as hot as can be tolerated. Cover the mush with another cloth. Leave the poultice on for one to two hours until dry. Repeat four times a day until the boil comes to a head and drains spontaneously.

Pork Poultice

Salt pork or bacon poultices are commonly used to treat various skin afflictions throughout New England and Appalachia. To treat a boil, you can try using a pork poultice. The poultice does not need to be hot, but the meat used should be fat meat. It is probably the constituents in the fat and the salt used to preserve the meat that bring the boil to a head.

DIRECTIONS: Roll some fatty pork or bacon in salt and place the meat between two pieces of cloth. Apply the poultice to the boil. Repeat throughout the day until the boil comes to a head and drains.

DIRECTIONS: Hard boil an egg. Crack off the shell and carefully peel the outer skin off the egg. Wet it and apply the egg skin directly to the boil and cover with a clean cloth.

Boils & Carbuncles

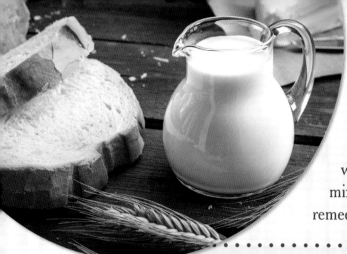

Bread & Milk Poultice

Poultices made of bread and milk have been used to treat boils in New England, Appalachia, Indiana, and among Hispanics in southwestern Colorado. It is the drawing nature of the mixture and the heat of the poultice that make this remedy work.

DIRECTIONS: Heat one cup of milk and slowly add three teaspoons of salt. Simmer the mixture for ten minutes. Thicken the mixture by adding flour or crumbled bread pieces. Divide the mixture into four poultices and apply one poultice to the boil every half hour. The poultice may also be applied before bedtime, held in place with a cloth, and kept on overnight.

Burdock

Burdock (*Arctium lappa, A. minus*) is considered a universal remedy for treating boils in contemporary European and North American herbalism. Drinking burdock tea to treat boils is a remedy still practiced today in Appalachia and in parts of rural Indiana. The constituents in burdock bring circulation to the surface of the skin and induce a light sweat. This increased circulation and corresponding movement of fluid and lymph at the surface of the skin may be responsible for the treatment's healing effect.

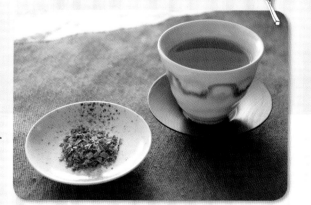

DIRECTIONS: Place one ounce of dried and ground burdock root in one quart of water. Bring to a boil and simmer on low heat for thirty minutes. Drink four cups of the hot tea each day until the boil comes to a head and drains. Along with this remedy, you can apply a poultice of fresh boiled burdock leaves directly to the boil.

Nutmeg

A popular remedy for treating boils in New England, Appalachia, and parts of the American Southwest is eating nutmeg (*Myristica fragrans*). Nutmeg is also sometimes applied directly to the boil as a poultice. Nutmeg stimulates the body's circulation, which conceivably could assist the body in fighting the infection of the boil.

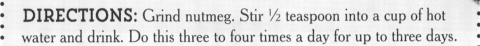

DIRECTIONS: Grind nutmeg. Stir ½ teaspoon into a cup of hot water and drink. Do this three to four times a day for up to three days.

Chrysanthemum Flowers

Drinking chrysanthemum flower tea is a Chinese remedy for treating boils that is still used in contemporary Chinese medicine today. The tea may also be applied as a compress. Chrysanthemum (*Chrysanthemum indicum flos*) flower tea is a common beverage among Asians in the United States and can usually be purchased in any Chinese or Korean food or herb shop. The Chinese name for the tea (and the herb) is *yeh-chu-hua*. Chinese and Japanese researchers have found constituents in chrysanthemum tea that inhibit *Staphylococcus* bacteria, the strain of bacteria that causes boils.

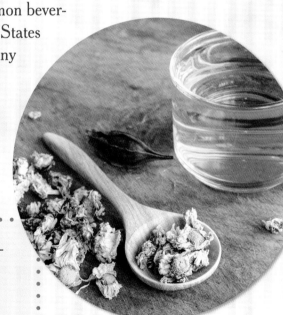

DIRECTIONS: Brew chrysanthemum flower tea according to the directions on the package. Dip a cloth in the hot tea and apply it to the boil every one to two hours. You can also drink three to four cups of the tea each day.

Boils & Carbuncles

BURNS & SUNBURNS

Although they can be quite painful, many burns are minor.

Burns are medically classified in two ways: by the depth of the burn and by the amount of body area the burn covers. Deep burns and burns covering large surface areas require medical examination. The most superficial burn is the first-degree burn, which is typical of a simple sunburn. A second-degree burn penetrates deeper into the skin and is usually accompanied by blisters. Third-degree burns involve deep tissue destruction. Third-degree burns may not blister, so they at first may appear to be less serious than they are. Often the skin looks whitish or charred. The chief risk of second- and third-degree burns is infection, and the more surface area that is affected, the more serious the risk. Infection may enter through ruptured blisters or through seemingly intact skin that has been burned. Many remedies are inappropriate for these burns, and some could actually promote infection. Conventional treatment for simple superficial burns includes cooling the tissues as soon as possible to reduce inflammation and blistering, and applying soothing ointments. This is the same strategy used by healers throughout the world. Some of the natural remedies below, such as aloe vera and plantain leaf, are disinfectants and probably helped to save lives endangered by infected burns in the past.

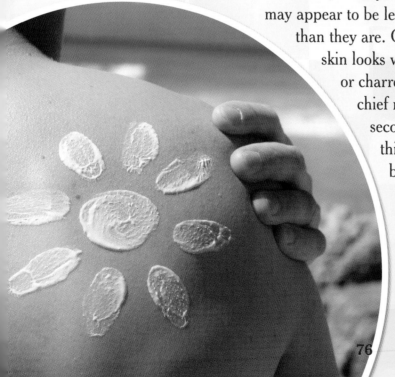

Remedies for
BURNS & SUNBURNS

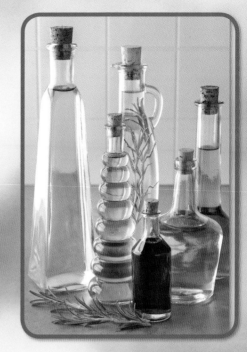

Vinegar

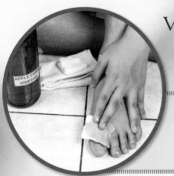

Vinegar washes are recommended in natural remedies from New England and New Mexico. Vinegar is both astringent and antiseptic, and like cool water, it helps to prevent blisters.

Directions: Apply vinegar to the burn every few minutes. Dilute the vinegar if the skin is very sensitive.

Tobacco

An American Indian treatment for burns is to wash the area in tobacco tea. Indiana medical folklore suggests applying a wad of chewing tobacco to the burned area.

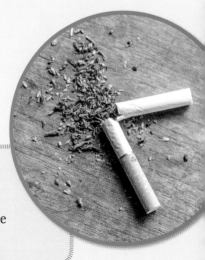

Directions: Remove the tobacco from a package of cigarettes and add it to one quart of water. Boil the water until the volume is reduced to one pint. Strain and let cool to room temperature. Wash the burn area with the tea as often as you'd like.

Aloe Vera

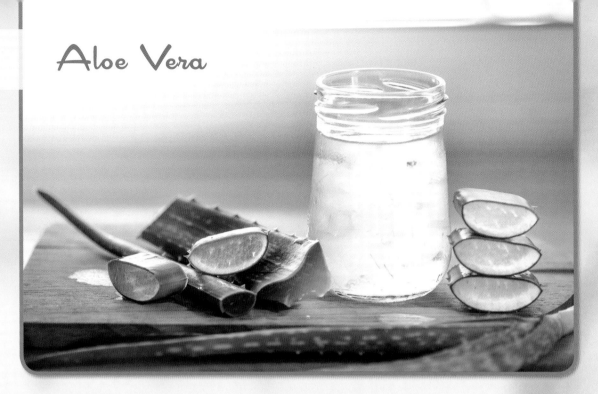

The juice of the aloe vera plant has been used as a burn remedy by practically every culture. Aloe vera is recommended as a remedy for burns—from sunburn to serious third-degree burns—in the literature of American Indians, New Englanders, the Amish, Indiana residents, the Romani, residents of northern Georgia, and Chinese immigrants. Aloe vera gel also acts as a disinfectant and reduces bacteria in burns.

Directions: For a small burn, break off a leaf, slice it down the middle, and rub the gel on the skin. To make a poultice of aloe, place the cut leaf on the burned area, and wrap the area with gauze. You can also apply store-bought aloe gel or juice. An alternate formula is to extend the aloe vera sap with olive oil. Here's how: Add eight ounces of extra virgin olive oil to two ounces of fresh squeezed aloe vera sap. Apply directly to the burn area.

Honey

Honey is a universal natural remedy to disinfect wounds and burns throughout the world. It is highly regarded in the literature of the Amish, Chinese immigrants, Indiana residents, and residents of the American Southwest. Honey naturally attracts water, and, when applied to a burn or wound, draws fluids out of the tissues, effectively cleaning the wound. Furthermore, most bacteria cannot live in the presence of honey. Honey is sometimes applied to gauze and used to dress severe burns in conventional medicine. In the early 1990s, physicians at a hospital in Maharashtra, India, performed clinical trials comparing honey-impregnated gauze with three different conventional burn treatments, and the honey treatment was superior in each case.

In a 1991 study, the doctors compared the honey-gauze to gauze treated with silver sulfadiazine. In fifty-two patients treated with honey, ninety-one percent of wounds were sterile within seven days. In the fifty-two patients treated with silver sulfadiazine, ninety-three percent of wounds still showed signs of infection after seven days. The burns of the honey-treated patients began to heal in seven days, while for the other group, healing began on average in thirteen days. Of the wounds treated with honey, eighty-seven percent healed within fifteen days; only ten percent of the wounds healed in the control group during that time. Important: The honey also provided greater pain relief and resulted in less scarring.

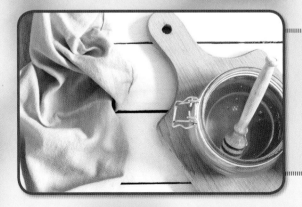

Directions: Apply honey to a piece of sterile gauze, and place directly on the burn, honey side to the skin. Change the dressing three to four times a day. Be sure to seek medical attention for serious burns.

COLD & FLU

The common cold is aptly named. It is so common, in fact, that all human beings from every region of the globe experience it at one time or another during their lives.

A simple common cold is a collection of familiar symptoms signaling an infection of the upper respiratory tract, which includes the nose, throat, and sinuses. At least five major categories of viruses cause colds. One of these groups, and perhaps the most common, the rhinoviruses, includes a minimum of 100 different viruses. The viruses that cause a cold reproduce in the mucous membranes. The viruses do not penetrate deeper into the body—into the gastrointestinal tract, for example—because they cannot survive at the higher body temperatures there.

Although we often say "colds and flu" in the same breath, influenza is a very different disease from the common cold. The influenza virus takes up residence mainly in the throat and bronchial tract. If you have the flu, you usually have a fever, and a fever is not usually present in a cold. The fever usually passes within three days, but the fatigue, muscle aches, and cough that result from the flu can linger for weeks. Influenza will not seriously injure a normally healthy person, but those with preexisting lung conditions, the elderly, and others with weakened resis-

tance are especially prone to the flu's deadly effects.

Flu is known as the "Last of the Great Plagues" because it kills so many people worldwide each year, including about 20,000 Americans. And when highly virulent flu strains periodically erupt, the death toll can rise even higher. For example, a flu epidemic just after World War I killed more than 30 million people worldwide.

The conventional treatment for flu in those at high risk for fatal complications is immunization in late fall with a flu vaccine. Immunization is also recommended for those who care for such high-risk patients. The antiviral drug ribavarin can be taken as well; it may be effective in preventing severe pneumonia caused by the influenza virus.

Some patients request antibiotics from their doctors to treat a cold or flu episode, and unfortunately, many doctors comply. Antibiotic drugs are good only for bacterial infections and are ineffective against colds and flu. In fact, taking them inappropriately may promote the development of drug-resistant bacterial strains and may render the antibiotics ineffective later on when the patient really needs them. The drug resistant strains can also be passed on to others.

Aspirin and other pain-killing drugs are also inappropriate treatments for cold and flu. Even though they may provide some temporary relief, they may suppress the immune system and can actually prolong the infection. And giving aspirin to children for colds and flu is a no-no. In rare cases, it can lead to the development of Reye syndrome, a serious and often fatal neurological disorder.

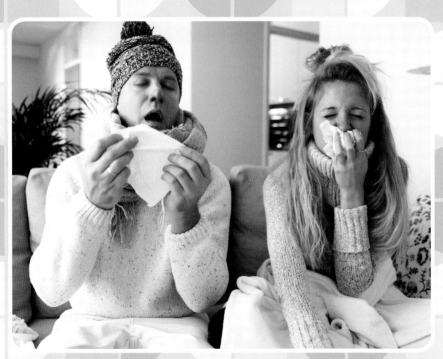

SWEATING IT OUT

Sweating is essential to cooling the body during a fever. Many traditional remedies use herbs for this purpose. These diaphoretic herbs have constituents that, when eaten, increase the blood circulation to the skin, which causes perspiration and ultimately lowers the fever.

It is essential to drink plenty of fluids when taking these herbs, however, or dehydration may result. Elder, ginger, yarrow, mint, boneset, pennyroyal, thyme, horsemint, beebalm, lemon balm, catnip, and garlic are all diaphoretic herbs. They're most effective when taken as hot teas. After drinking the tea, go to bed, wrap up in warm blankets, and sweat it out. Continue to drink plenty of fluids.

Remedies for
THE COLD & FLU

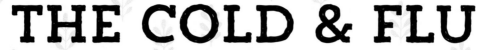

Echinacea

Echinacea (*Echinacea angustifolia, Echinacea purpurea*) is, without a doubt, the most commonly used natural remedy for treating colds and flu in the United States today. In fact, echinacea is the best selling medicinal herb in the country.

Echinacea was used as a remedy by the American Indians of the Great Plains states. The tribes residing in those areas used the herb for all manner of infectious diseases. Eclectic physicians, a now-defunct North American school of doctors who used herbs as medicines, adopted the use of echinacea in the mid-1880s. By 1920, it was the remedy they prescribed the most. The use of echinacea spread to Germany in the 1930s, where it remains an approved medicine today—used to treat colds, flu, and other conditions related to underlying deficiencies of the immune system.

Echinacea is also famous in the contemporary medical herbalism of Britain, Australia, and North America for its ability to "abort" a cold or flu. German clinical trials show that echinacea, taken preventively during cold and flu season, can reduce the frequency and severity of a viral infection. In fact, if echinacea is taken at the first onset of symptoms, the cold may never develop at all. Once a cold has set in, however, the other remedies in the section may be more beneficial.

Directions: Purchase a tincture of echinacea at a health food store, herb shop, or drugstore. At the first sign of a cold or flu, take one teaspoon of the tincture every hour for three hours. If the infection persists, take one dropperful every three hours.

Elder Flowers

Elderberry comprises about thirteen species of deciduous shrubs native to North America and Europe. European settlers brought elderberry plants with them to the American colonies. The Paiute and Shoshone Indians in the Rocky Mountain region used the leaves and flowers of a North American species of elderberry to treat colds, flu, and fevers.

A tea made of elderberry flowers is approved by the German government as a medicine for colds, especially if a cough is present. The flower tea is also used to treat colds and flu in the natural medicine of contemporary Indiana. The Michigan Amish use the tea as well.

Recent research in Israel and Panama has shown that elderberry juice stimulates the immune system and also directly inhibits the influenza virus. Constituents in the plant's flowers

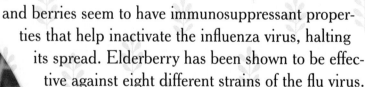

Directions: Place ½ ounce of elderberry flowers in a one-quart canning jar and fill with boiling water. Cover and let steep for twenty minutes. Strain and pour a cup of the tea. Sweeten with honey. Take one cup once every four hours when you have a cold or flu. Wrap yourself up in warm blankets after drinking the tea to help induce sweating.

and berries seem to have immunosuppressant properties that help inactivate the influenza virus, halting its spread. Elderberry has been shown to be effective against eight different strains of the flu virus. Drinking too much elderberry tea, more than indicated in the directions below, however, can leave you feeling nauseous. And, because of a documented diuretic effect, prolonged use may result in hypokalemia, or potassium loss. Avoid the use of elder during pregnancy and lactation.

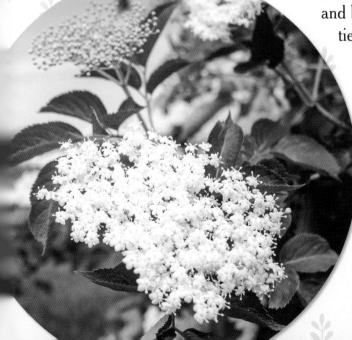

83

Boneset

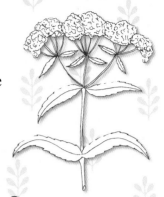

The herb boneset (*Eupatorium perfoliatum*) got its name during an influenza epidemic in Pennsylvania in the 1700s. The flu was called "breakbone fever"; the word *breakbone* referred to the muscle aches and pains that accompanied the virus. Taking the herb, however, proved to "set the bones" and relieve the aches. The colonists learned the use of the plant from the Cherokee and Iroquois Indians and other eastern American Indian tribes.

The use of boneset for treating colds and flu spread to Europe. Today, some German medical schools continue to study its use. Boneset is frequently prescribed in Germany for treating acute viral infections, for which antibiotic drugs are not effective. The herb also continues to be used today in the natural medicine traditions of Indiana and southern Illinois.

Constituents have been identified in boneset that are both immune-stimulating and anti-inflammatory. Do not overdo it with boneset, however, because it can induce vomiting if taken in large quantities. It was actually used for that purpose in the 18th and 19th centuries. Boneset is also know to have constituents that are allergenic. Boneset should be avoided during pregnancy and lactation.

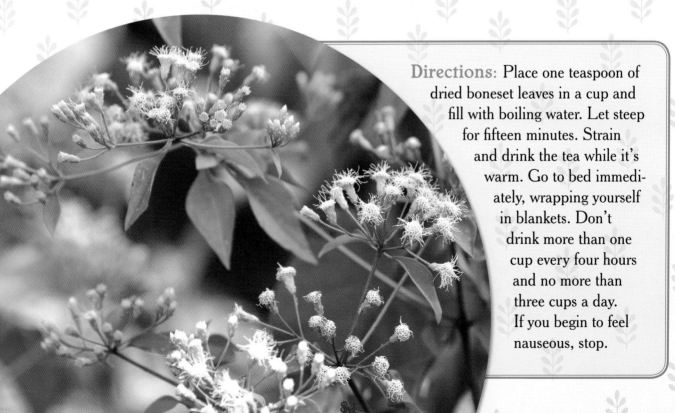

Directions: Place one teaspoon of dried boneset leaves in a cup and fill with boiling water. Let steep for fifteen minutes. Strain and drink the tea while it's warm. Go to bed immediately, wrapping yourself in blankets. Don't drink more than one cup every four hours and no more than three cups a day. If you begin to feel nauseous, stop.

Yarrow

The ancient Greeks used yarrow (*Achillea millefolium*) as a remedy for colds, flu, and fever. At least eighteen American Indian tribes from all corners of North America used yarrow for the same purpose. The early colonists throughout North America used yarrow as a household medicine for a wide variety of ailments, usually conditions that were infectious or inflammatory in nature. The use of yarrow tea for colds and flu survives today in the medicine of North Carolina, Indiana, and upstate New York. Yarrow has documented anti-inflammatory, antispasmodic, diuretic, mild sedative, and moderate antibacterial activities.

Directions: Place one ounce of dried or fresh yarrow in a one-quart canning jar. Fill the jar with boiling water and cover tightly. Let steep for twenty minutes. Strain, pour, and sweeten with honey. Take three cups a day, bundling up in blankets and resting in bed after each cup.

Ginger

Ginger tea is a cold remedy mentioned in the literature of New England, Appalachia, North Carolina, Indiana, and even China. Ginger induces sweating, which helps to cool the body during fever. Ginger contains twelve different aromatic anti-inflammatory compounds, including some with aspirin-like effects. Its other proven actions result from its antinauseant and antivertigo properties. Ginger also has carminative (gas relieving), diaphoretic (sweat inducing), and antispasmodic activities.

Directions: Cut a fresh ginger root (about the size of your thumb) into thin slices. Place the slices in one quart of water. Bring to a boil. Cover the pot and simmer on the lowest possible heat for thirty minutes. Let cool for thirty minutes more. Strain and drink ½ to one cup three to five times a day. Sweeten with honey, as desired.

Cold & Flu

Peppermint

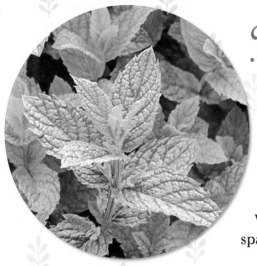

Peppermint (*Mentha piperita*) is a natural remedy used in Indiana to treat colds. Cornmint (*Mentha arvensis*), a close relative of the plant, is used in China for the same purpose. Both plants, when taken as a hot tea, induce sweating and help to cool a fever. Also, the essential oils in the plants, including menthol, act as decongestants when drunk as a tea or inhaled. Peppermint also has anti-spasmodic and carminative properties.

Directions: Place ½ ounce of peppermint leaves in a one-quart jar. Fill the jar with boiling water and cover tightly. Let steep twenty minutes. Strain the liquid and drink two or three cups a day. Wrap yourself in blankets and rest in bed after each cup.

Horsemint-Beebalm Tea

Two closely related species, horsemint (*Monarda punctata*) and beebalm (*Monarda menthaefolia, M. didyma*), are used in natural medicine similarly to the way thyme is used. (Horsemint is native to the eastern United States; beebalm to the Rocky Mountains.) Both plants, like thyme, contain high amounts of the constituent thymol, which acts as an expectorant and antiseptic. Both plants also induce sweating and can help cool a fever.

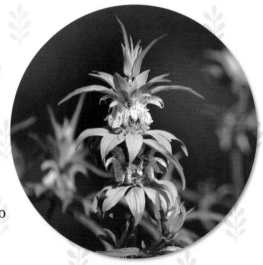

Directions: Put one teaspoon of dried leaves of either plant in a cup and fill with boiling water. Let steep for five minutes while inhaling the fumes through both the nose and mouth. Strain, sweeten with honey, and sip the tea slowly. Do this three to five times a day.

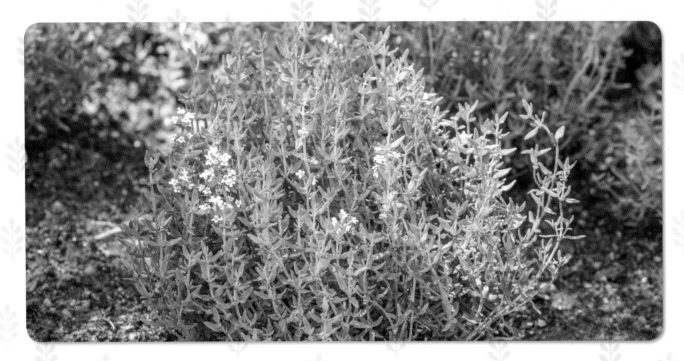

Thyme

Thyme tea (*Thymus vulgaris*) is recommended as a treatment for cold or flu in the natural medicine of Indiana and China. Thyme taken in the form of a hot tea also induces sweating and helps to cool a fever. In addition, its constituent oil, thymol, is a powerful expectorant and antiseptic. The constituent readily disperses in the steam of a hot tea. Inhaling the steam may effectively spread the thymol throughout the mucous membranes of the upper respiratory tract and bronchial tree. Thus, thymol may help inhibit bacteria, viruses, or fungi from infecting the membranes. Thyme also has mild analgesic and antipyretic (fever reducing) properties.

This remedy from Indiana suggests sipping the tea slowly while inhaling its fragrance. In China, the same method is used as a preventive—for when colds or flu are "going around."

Directions:
Put one teaspoon of dried thyme leaves in a cup and fill with boiling water. Let steep for five minutes while inhaling the fumes through both the nose and mouth. Then, strain the tea, sweeten with honey, and sip slowly. Go to bed and bundle up warmly in blankets.

Lemon Balm

Several Indiana residents responding to a poll of natural remedies in the 1980s recommended lemon balm (*Melissa officinalis*) tea for cold and flu. The plant, which is native to southern Europe and northern Africa, now grows throughout North America as well. Lemon balm has long been used as a relaxing and sweat-inducing herb. The 12th century German mystic and healer Hildegarde von Bingen stated, "Lemon balm contains within it the virtues of a dozen other plants."

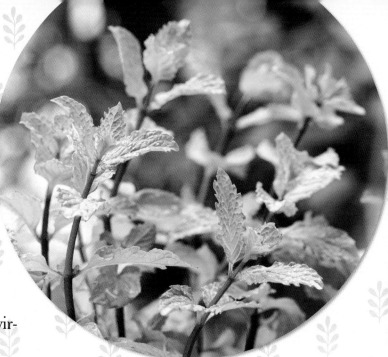

Lemon balm is approved today by the German government as a medicine for digestive complaints and sleeping disorders, though it is not recommended specifically for colds or flu.

Its aromatic oils contain anti-viral compounds that may help disinfect the mucous membranes, however. Of the sweat-inducing herbs included in this section, lemon balm is probably the mildest and the most suitable for use in children. Lemon balm is also a mild sedative and can help relax a restless patient suffering from cold or flu.

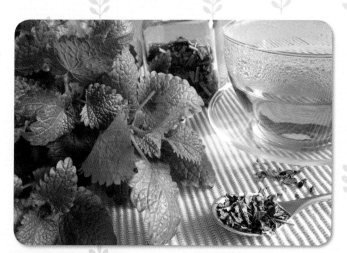

Directions: Place one teaspoon of the dried herb in a cup and fill with boiling water. Let steep for ten minutes. Inhale the steam from the cup. Strain and drink up to four cups a day. Sweeten with honey as desired.

Garlic

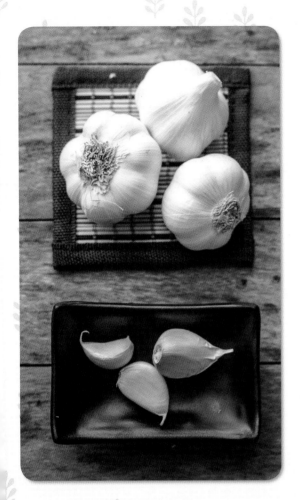

The recommendation to take garlic for colds comes from New England, the American Southwest, and all the way from China. Garlic has been used for colds, bronchial problems, and fevers in cultures throughout the world since the dawn of written medical history—even the ancient Egyptians used it to treat cough and fever.

Garlic's constituents are antibacterial, antiviral, and antifungal. Garlic also stimulates the immune system, increasing the body's resistance to invaders. In addition, garlic is an expectorant and induces sweating, helping to reduce fever. Garlic has been approved as a medicine for colds and coughs and a variety of other illnesses by the pharmaceutical regulatory commission of the European Union, a confederation of modern European nations that has dropped trade barriers and is working toward economic regulation and a common currency. Garlic can also lower cholesterol and thin the blood. Note that garlic taken in high doses can irritate the stomach.

Directions: Blend three cloves of garlic in a blender with a little water. (A clove must be cut or crushed in order to release its constituents.) If you want, add half a lemon, skin and all, to the garlic. Put the contents in a cup and fill the cup with boiling water. Let steep for five minutes, inhaling the fragrance. Strain, add honey, and drink the entire cup in sips. Do this two to three times a day while you have a cold or flu or once a day to prevent infection during epidemics.

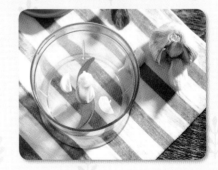

Alternately, peel and chop three whole garlic bulbs and soak them in one pint of wine (red or white) in a closed container for a month. Shake the jar once a day. Then, strain and take one tablespoon of the wine each day as a preventive measure.

Onions

Onions are used to treat colds in virtually every folk tradition in North America—whether eaten raw, roasted, or boiled; taken in the form of teas, milk, or wine; worn in a sock or in a bag around the neck; or applied to the chest as a poultice. Wild onions have been used for the same purpose by American Indian tribes in every region of the country. Using onions to treat colds continues today in the natural medicine of New England, upstate New York, North Carolina, Appalachia, Indiana, and within Chinese cultures throughout North America.

The constituents in onions—the same that cause onion's volatile vapors to burn the eyes—are antimicrobial. Onions also have expectorant qualities, which induce the flow of healthy cleansing mucous. Onions induce sweating as well, helping to cool a fever.

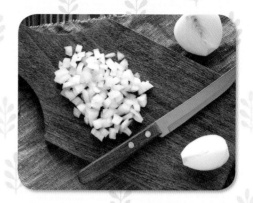

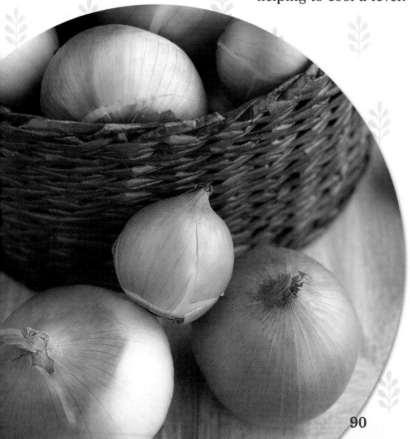

Directions: Cut up one whole large onion and simmer in a covered pot for twenty minutes. Strain if desired to remove pulp. Drink a cup of the tea three to four times daily when you have a cold or flu.

Alternately, try chewing raw onions—but don't swallow until the onions are thoroughly chewed. Note: Chewing too many onions can cause your stomach to become irritated.

To make an onion poultice for chest colds, slice three large onions, discarding the outer paper-like skin. Cover with water and simmer for twenty minutes. Strain. Layer the cooked onions between two cloths. Apply to the chest for twenty to thirty minutes.

90

Sage

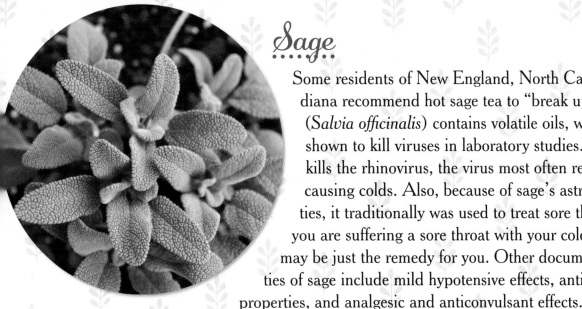

Some residents of New England, North Carolina, and Indiana recommend hot sage tea to "break up" a cold. Sage (*Salvia officinalis*) contains volatile oils, which have been shown to kill viruses in laboratory studies. It specifically kills the rhinovirus, the virus most often responsible for causing colds. Also, because of sage's astringent qualities, it traditionally was used to treat sore throats. So, if you are suffering a sore throat with your cold, hot sage tea may be just the remedy for you. Other documented properties of sage include mild hypotensive effects, anti-inflammatory properties, and analgesic and anticonvulsant effects.

Directions: Place one teaspoon of sage in a cup and fill with boiling water. Cover and let steep for ten minutes. Strain, add a little lemon and honey, and drink.

Repeat three to four times a day for as long as you have a cold.

Vinegar

A cold remedy from Indiana calls for inhaling the fumes of vinegar. This remedy is as old as ancient Greece—the Greek physician Hippocrates recommended the treatment for coughs and respiratory infections. Vinegar is a weak acid. Inhaling its fumes changes the acidity of the mucous membranes in the upper respiratory tract, making the membranes inhospitable to viruses. Due to its acidic nature, avoid splashing vinegar into the eyes or onto cuts.

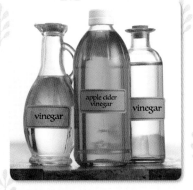

Directions: In a jar, pour ½ cup of boiling water over ½ cup of vinegar. Gently inhale the steam. Be careful not to burn yourself.

Cold & Flu

Lemon

The contemporary natural remedies of New England and Indiana call for drinking "hot lemonade" during a cold or flu. The practice is at least as old as the ancient Romans.

Lemon juice, like vinegar, is acidic. Drinking it helps to acidify the mucous membranes, making the membranes inhospitable to bacteria or viruses. Lemon oil, which gives the juice its fragrance, is like a pharmacy in itself—it contains antibacterial, antiviral, antifungal, and anti-inflammatory constituents. Five of the constituents are specifically active against the influenza virus. Lemon oil is also an expectorant, increasing the flow of healthy mucous. And lemon is very tasty—its flavor is used to promote compliance in taking cold and flu products.

Directions: Place one chopped whole lemon—skin, pulp, and all—in a pot and add one cup of boiling water. While letting the mixture steep for five minutes, inhale the fumes. Then, strain and drink. Do this at the onset of a cold, and repeat three to four times a day for the duration of the cold.

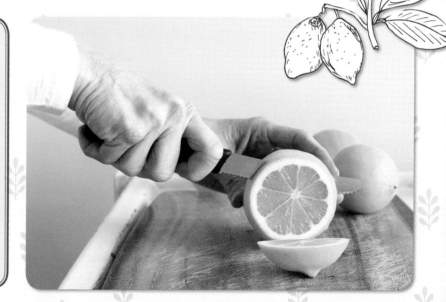

Mustard Plaster

The mustard plaster has been used medicinally in Europe at least since the time of the ancient Romans. The contemporary Amish still recommend it for treating chest colds and bronchitis. It works mainly by increasing circulation, perspiration, and heat in the afflicted area. In addition, when its irritant antimicrobial and anti-inflammatory volatile substances are inhaled, mustard may also have a medicinal effect on the mucous membranes of the upper respiratory tract. The active principle is allylisothiocyanate, which is also present in horseradish and watercress.

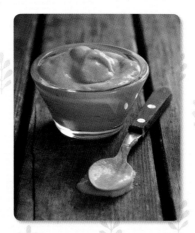

Directions: Mix ½ cup mustard with one cup flour. Stir warm water into the mustard and flour mixture until a paste is formed. This allows for the active principle to be released. Spread the mixture on a piece of cotton or muslin that has been soaked in hot water. Cover with a second piece of dry material. Lay the moist side of the poultice across the person's chest or back. Leave the poultice on for fifteen to thirty minutes. Remove promptly if the person experiences any discomfort. (Be careful not to blister or burn the skin. You may want to lift the cloth every five minutes or so to see how red the skin is.)

Vaporize It

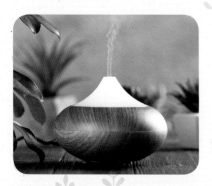

The contemporary Amish suggest using a vaporizer and adding essential oils to the water, such as pine, cedar, or mint. Many of the aromatic constituents of these plants have antimicrobial properties. If you can smell the aroma, then at least a small amount of the constituent has reached your mucous membranes and may assist in killing viruses there. Peppermint oil also contains menthol, which acts as a decongestant. Excessive inhalation can be hazardous to sensitive or allergic young children, however.

Directions: Add a few drops of essential oils to the water of a commercial vaporizer. If you've purchased concentrated essential oils, be sure to dilute them with at least five parts of a carrier oil (such as almond oil) before adding them to the water. Place the vaporizer next to the sick bed and keep it running around the clock.

CONSTIPATION

Regularity is actually a relative term. What matters is not the frequency of your bowel movements, but whether your normal routine alters.

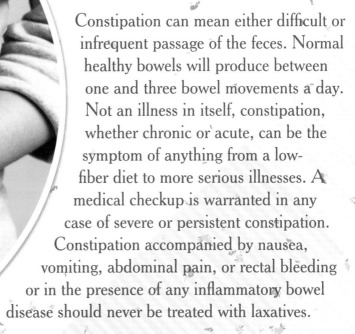

Constipation can mean either difficult or infrequent passage of the feces. Normal healthy bowels will produce between one and three bowel movements a day. Not an illness in itself, constipation, whether chronic or acute, can be the symptom of anything from a low-fiber diet to more serious illnesses. A medical checkup is warranted in any case of severe or persistent constipation. Constipation accompanied by nausea, vomiting, abdominal pain, or rectal bleeding or in the presence of any inflammatory bowel disease should never be treated with laxatives.

The most common cause of constipation in modern society is the modern diet. Constipation is classified by medical anthropologists H.C. Trowell and D.P. Burkitt as a "Western" condition, meaning that the condition does not appear in primitive people eating traditional diets—that is, until Western foods, such as sugar, white flour, and canned goods, are added.

Conventional physicians, alternative doctors, and natural healers alike all warn against the use of strong laxatives to force a bowel movement. From a medical point of view, if the constipation is due to a serious underlying disease, the laxative can cause injury and make that condition worse. Chronic use of strong laxatives also creates "laxative dependence"—a condition in which the bowels become so exhausted that they can no longer provide a normal bowel movement without the stimulation of more laxatives. Laxative dependence can also cause electrolyte (such as sodium and potassium) imbalances.

Conventional treatment for constipation, after a thorough investigation of the cause, is to increase fiber and liquids in the diet and to administer bulk laxatives (also called stool softeners) such as psyllium husks. An increase in fruits and vegetables in the diet is also encouraged. Eat six or more servings of vegetables each day.

Many of the remedies for treating constipation include herbs that act as strong laxatives, but their use for more than seven to ten days is not warranted. Anything stronger than a bulk laxative is contraindicated in pregnancy, however, because the same constituents that make the colon wall contract to produce a bowel movement can make the uterus contract as well. Stimulating laxatives are also contraindicated for use in children under twelve years of age.

Castor Oil

A suggestion from the natural medicine of contemporary Indiana is to rub warm castor oil on a colicky baby's stomach and keep the baby covered with warm clothes. (Castor oil taken internally is a strong laxative, and it should never be given to a baby or a child.) The external use of castor oil for digestive pain and complaints gained great popularity in North American healing traditions in the late 20th century, thanks to the teachings of mystic Edgar Cayce. (Cayce, an American Christian, was known for giving medical advice, often while in a trance-like state. His books remain popular today.) Cayce claimed that castor oil improved the functioning of the gut's immune system. No scientific evidence exists to support the claim, but the practice continues and appears to be harmless.

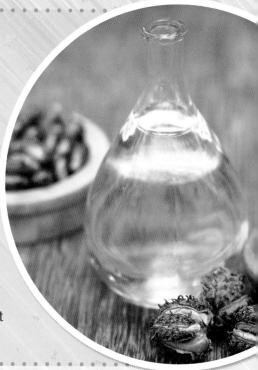

Remedies for
CONSTIPATION

Senna

Well-known as a laxative, senna leaves *(Cassia senna)*, most of which are imported from India, were brought to this country by European colonists. A North American variety of senna was used in the same way by Indians in eastern parts of the United States. Senna leaves have been used as a laxative by the Amish. Senna has been used for the same purpose in the natural medicine of New England, Appalachia, and the Southwest. Senna is also a component of some over-the-counter laxatives in North America and Europe. Senna is contraindicated in children, during pregnancy, and for more than ten days at a time.

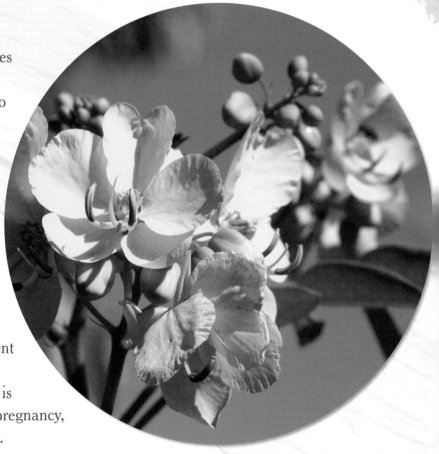

Directions: Do not use excessive amounts of senna. Place ¼ to ½ teaspoon of the dried crushed leaves or powder in a cup and fill with boiling water. Let steep seven to ten minutes. (A full teaspoon in a cup of tea is strong enough to produce abdominal cramping.)

Epsom Salts

Epsom salts are composed of magnesium sulfate. The salt was first prepared from the waters of mineral springs in Epsom, England, where it was discovered in 1695. Their use as a commercial laxative spread quickly in the medicine of Europe; the salts remain popular there today. Epsom salts are now produced industrially and not from the springs in Epsom. The salts act as a laxative by drawing water out of the body and into the intestine. Epsom salts are listed in the medicine of New England and are widely used throughout North America as an over-the-counter laxative. Habitual use can cause dehydration and laxative dependence, however, so don't use Epsom salts for more than seven days.

Directions: Place two or three teaspoons of Epsom salts in a glass of warm water and drink. Do this once a day.

Flax Seed

Flax seed (*Linum usitatissimum*) is a New England remedy for treating constipation. The remedy is also used among the Amish and by some Romani. Flax is a bulk laxative, meaning that its fiber absorbs water, expands, and provides bulk for bowel movements. Flax seed also contains high amounts of essential fatty acids. Flax seed works in the same way as psyllium seed, the chief component of the commercial bulk laxative Metamucil.

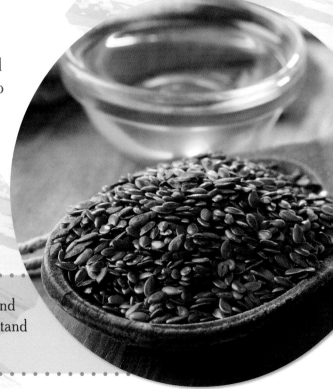

Directions: Take two teaspoons of flax seeds. Grind them and add to an eight-ounce glass of water. Let stand for half an hour and drink, seeds and all.

Constipation

A Romani Formula

The following formula, related by a Spanish Gypsy in Wanja von Hausen's *Gypsy Folk Medicine*, combines several laxative substances with herbs to reduce tension and improve digestion. Note the absence of any strong laxatives, making it a safe formula for regular use.

Directions: Mix a half-handful of rosemary blossoms or leaves and a handful of black elderberries in a pint of extra-virgin olive oil. Shake well and store for three days in a cool, dark place.

Crush one tablespoon of flax seeds in a coffee grinder or with a mortar and pestle. Place the crushed seeds in a bowl, adding the olive oil and herb mixture. Crush two tablespoons of valerian root and add to the mixture. Place the entire mixture in a jar, shake well, and store for seven days, shaking it once or twice a day. Strain the oil through cheesecloth or gauze, and store in a cool, dark place. Take one tablespoon first thing in the morning on an empty stomach. If needed, take a second tablespoon in the evening before dinner. Keep taking the oil until your bowel movements are regular.

Boneset

In colonial days, boneset (*Eupatorium perfoliatum*) was one of the most often used medicinal herbs in North America. Ethnobotanical sources say that it was found hanging in the houses or barns of every "well regulated" household in the colonies. Hot boneset tea was taken to treat fevers, colds, and flu. Cold boneset tea was taken as a digestive tonic, and sometimes, as a mild laxative.

The use of boneset as a laxative was recorded among the Mohawk Indians and persists today in the medicine of Appalachia. When using boneset, always use the dried leaves, however, because fresh boneset contains mildly toxic substances. And don't exceed the recommended amounts, because larger amounts can cause nausea or induce vomiting, one of its older medical uses.

Directions: Place one teaspoon of dried boneset leaves in a cup and fill with boiling water. Cover and let stand until cooled to room temperature. Drink ¼ cup three times a day for up to five days.

Sesame Seeds

According to the Amish, sesame seeds have a laxative effect. Chinese natural medicine claims the same. The seeds are nutritious and also contain about fifty-five percent oil, which helps to moisten the intestines in those suffering from dry constipation.

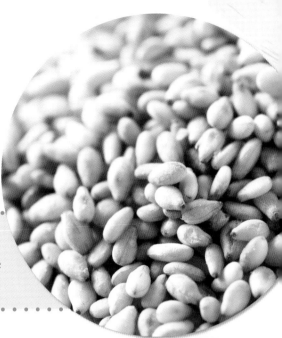

Directions: Eat up to ½ ounce of sesame seeds a day. Grind them fresh in a coffee grinder and sprinkle on food like a condiment.

Hot Water

A remedy from New England also mentioned by the Amish is to drink a cup of hot water in the morning. Similar practices, slightly modified, appear throughout the world. In the medicine of India, the prescription is to drink a quart of room temperature water in the morning. German followers of the water cures of Father Sebastian Kneipp take the water hot in one-tablespoon doses every half hour all day.

Drinking water in the morning to produce a bowel movement has a solid physiological basis. An internal digestive reflex causes the bowels to contract and move the stool in the direction of the anus in response to stretching of the stomach. The stretch reflex can be triggered most easily in the morning, when the stomach is most contracted. Drinking water can trigger this stretch reflex.

Directions: Drink one to three cups of hot water first thing in the morning on an empty stomach.

COUGHS

Coughing is more than an annoyance—it's a reflex that protects your breathing passages (including your lungs) from secretions that can clog them and hinder your intake of oxygen.

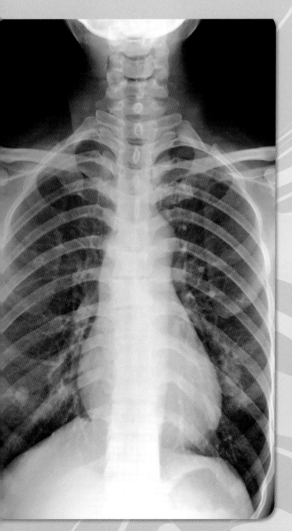

Coughing can result from inhaling dust, dirt, or irritating fumes; from breathing icy air; or from mistakenly drawing food into the airways. It can also be caused by mucus and other secretions from such respiratory disorders as the common cold, influenza, pneumonia, or tuberculosis.

The respiratory passages in the throat and lungs are constantly kept moist by a layer of mucus. This mucus traps small particles, viruses, bacteria, dust, pollen, or other materials. The surfaces of these passageways are so sensitive to touch that any irritation there will cause a cough reflex—a reflex that expels the irritating matter at velocities as high as 100 miles per hour. This reflex usually removes any loose mucus or other matter. A cough is thus a healthy healing mechanism, necessary to remove allergens, viruses, bacteria, or foreign matter from the respiratory tract.

Both pharmaceutical drugs and natural remedies aid coughs in several ways. Some remedies, like the herbs licorice or marshmallow, are demulcents; they moisten and soothe the throat and bronchial tract, reducing the cough reflex by reducing irritation of the tissues. Others, such as garlic or honey, are expectorants and work by promoting the secretion of fresh mucus, which aids the body in washing out irritants. Finally, cherry bark and the over-the-counter drug dextromethorphan, are respiratory sedatives. They act on the nervous system to reduce the cough reflex. Such a reduction is appropriate for short-term use when an unproductive cough interferes with sleep or is overly-exhausting. Sedatives are not appropriate for productive coughs with a lot of mucus, however, because the cough is necessary to clear the lungs of mucus.

According to the Public Citizen Health Research Group, dextromethorphan is the best cough suppressant to use. It is a component of many over-the-counter cough remedies and syrups. The Public Citizen Health Research Group recommends purchasing generic dextromethorphan at a pharmacy or taking a product containing only dextromethorphan, which will suppress a cough for about twelve hours and allow a good night's sleep.

The actions of cough remedies, even the over-the-counter pharmaceutical types, are difficult to prove. There is no scientific evidence supporting that these herbs effectively treat coughs, probably due to the difficulty in accurately measuring expectoration.

Coughs, Dry & Wet

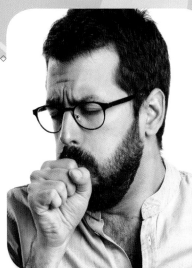

A cough is a healthy healing mechanism, necessary to remove allergens, viruses, or bacteria from the respiratory tract. Mucus traps these invading and irritating substances. The secretion of the mucus and its expulsion from your body when you cough is part of the body's healing process.

With some coughs—such as "wet" coughs—plenty of mucus is present, but the mucus is thick, gummy, and hard to expel. Acrid, irritating, and stimulating herbs are helpful for treating these types of coughs because they stimulate the flow of new clean mucus, which helps expel the old.

"Dry" coughs typically accompany the flu. Acrid and stimulating herbs only irritate dry coughs further because there is little mucus to expel. To treat a dry cough, try a soothing herb such as slippery elm, mallow, or licorice.

Remedies for COUGHS

Wild Cherry Bark

The use of wild cherry bark (*Prunus serotina*) to treat coughs was taught to the British colonists by the Cherokee and the Iroquois eastern Indian tribes. Other tribes throughout North America have used various wild cherry species in the same way. Use of the bark became very popular throughout the United States in the 19th century. Wild cherry bark is still used as a cough remedy in the medicine of the Amish, New Englanders, and residents of the Southwest. It is also used in contemporary North American and European medical herbalism. "Wild cherry" cough drops are available in stores today, although they are now made with artificial flavors instead of actual wild cherry bark.

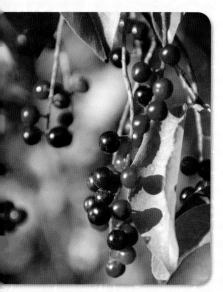

The bark's constituent prunasin reduces the cough reflex, so wild cherry is classified as a cough suppressant. Thus, it requires the same cautions as the over-the-counter medication dextromethorphan. Prunasin is a potentially toxic compound. But, if taken as a tea in the correct quantities, adults are safe using it. All cases of toxicity from wild cherry have occurred in children eating the fruit—called "choke cherries"—along with the toxic pits, which contain large amounts of prunasin and related compounds.

Wild cherry has expectorant and demulcent properties, too, so this herb is like a complete cough formula all rolled up in one. Wild cherry bark is especially suited to dry, irritating coughs. Combining it with another demulcent will further improve its effects.

Directions: Place one tablespoon of wild cherry bark and an equal part of licorice root in one pint of water. Boil for five minutes, remove from heat, sweeten with ½ cup of honey. Let stand until the mixture cools to room temperature. The dose is ¼ cup, no more than five times a day. To remain on the side of caution, don't give cherry bark to children under the age of twelve. Adults shouldn't take cherry bark for more than three consecutive days. Women should avoid cherry bark altogether if they are pregnant or nursing.

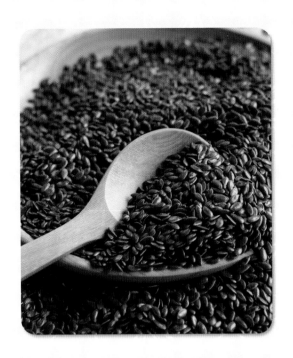

Flax Seed

New Englanders and residents of other eastern states use boiled flax seeds (*Linum usitatissimum*) to treat coughs. Boiled flax seeds make a thick demulcent that is soothing to the throat and bronchial tract.

Directions: Boil two or three tablespoons of flax seeds in one cup of water for a few minutes, until the water becomes gooey. Strain. Add equal parts of honey and lemon juice. For a dry irritable cough that's not producing much mucus, take one-tablespoon doses as needed.

Black Pepper

A remedy for coughs from New England, which also appears in Chinese folk medicine, is black pepper (*Piper nigrum*). The irritating properties of black pepper stimulate circulation and the flow of mucus. Black pepper works best on coughs producing a thick mucus; it is inappropriate for a dry, irritable cough with little expectoration.

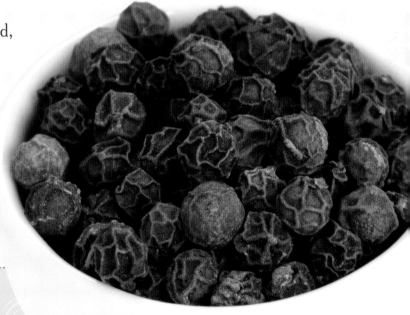

Directions: Place one teaspoon of black pepper and one tablespoon of honey in a cup and fill with boiling water. Let steep for ten to fifteen minutes. Take small sips as needed.

Coughs

Mustard Seed

An old New England cough remedy calls for mustard seed. Mustard is also used for treating coughs in the medicine of China. Mustard has irritating sulfur-containing compounds that stimulate the flow of mucus. Like pepper, above, it is only appropriate for congested productive coughs with plenty of mucus present. It will irritate a dry cough and make it worse.

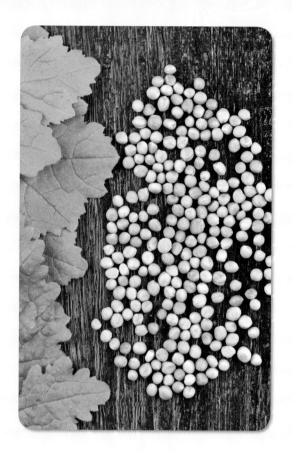

Directions: Crush one teaspoon of mustard seeds or grind them in a coffee grinder. Place the seeds in a cup and fill with warm water. Steep for fifteen minutes. (The expectorant compounds are not released until the mustard seeds are crushed or broken and allowed to sit in water or some other medium for about fifteen minutes.) Take in ¼-cup doses throughout the day.

Garlic

Early medical records from all over the globe show that garlic (*Allium sativum*) was used as a treatment for coughs and bronchial conditions. Garlic-honey syrups are standard cough treatments in the natural medicinal traditions of the Southwest today.

Garlic was acknowledged as an expectorant in the National Formulary of the United States from 1916 until 1936. Garlic is not appropriate for treating dry, unproductive coughs, however. It is best for treating coughs that are producing mucus.

Directions: Put one pound of sliced garlic in one quart of boiling water; let it soak for ten to twelve minutes, keeping the water warm (but not boiling). Strain and add four pounds of honey. Strain and bottle the syrup. When you feel congested, take one teaspoonful.

Onion Syrup

In *American Folk Medicine*, folklorist Clarence Meyer suggests taking a honey-and-onion syrup for treating coughs. Onions have anti-inflammatory properties that may reduce throat irritation, and honey is a natural expectorant, promoting the free flow of mucus. Onions also contain the antiviral constituent protocatechuic acid, which attacks viruses, including the one that may be causing the cough.

Directions: Chop six white onions and place them in a double boiler. Add ½ cup of honey and the juice of one lemon and cook at lowest heat possible for several hours. Strain the mixture and take by the tablespoon as needed—from every half an hour to every few hours.

Horehound

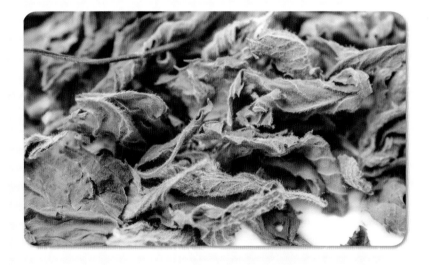

A remedy for coughs from contemporary New Mexico is horehound (*Marrubium vulgare*), a European plant that arrived in North America with both the Spanish and northern European colonists. Horehound has been used to treat coughs in European medicine since the time of the ancient Greeks. It was an official cough remedy in the United States Pharmacopoeia between 1840 and 1910, and it remains an approved medicine for coughs by the German government today.

Horehound stimulates the flow of mucus, and is indicated for use in moist unproductive coughs. It can be irritating and increase the discomfort of dry coughs, however.

Directions: Place one tablespoon of dried horehound in a cup and fill with boiling water. Cover and let steep for fifteen minutes. Sweeten with honey. Drink in ½-cup doses as often as desired.

Coughs

Osha Syrup

Osha (*Ligusticum porteri*) was a medicinal plant popular among American Indians and settlers residing in the higher elevations of the Rocky Mountains. Osha has a hot acrid taste, and its constituents possesses both expectorant and antiviral properties. American Indians of the area believed that osha has the power to repel evil spirits.

Directions: Grind one ounce of osha root in a coffee grinder. Heat one pint of honey in a pot, and add the osha root. Simmer slowly until the honey becomes thick. Leave the root in the honey and let cool to room temperature. Do not strain. Take one-tablespoon doses of the syrup four to six times a day as desired.

Mullein

Did you know you can make a cough syrup with the leaves of the mullein plant? Mullein (*Verbascum thapsus*) came to North America with the European colonists and is now naturalized throughout the United States and Canada. Its use as a cough medicine was quickly adopted by several American Indian tribes, including the Mohegan, Delaware, Cherokee, Creek, and Navaho. It appears today in the medicine of Appalachia and the Southwest. Mullein was an official cough medicine in the United States Pharmacopoeia from 1888 until 1936 and remains an approved medicine for cough in Germany. Recent research shows that mullein tea also may have an antiviral effect against the influenza virus.

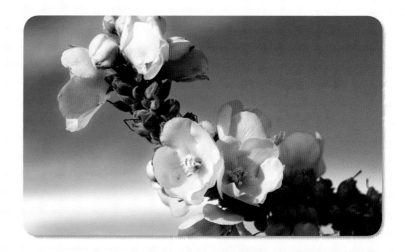

Directions: Place ½ pound of mullein leaves in a one-quart jar. Fill with boiling water and let cool to room temperature. Strain and add honey until the mixture has the consistency of a syrup. The dose is one tablespoon as needed.

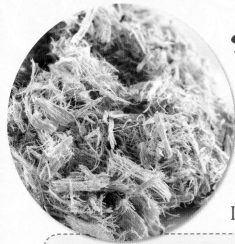

Slippery Elm

Slippery elm bark (*Ulmus fulva*) has a slimy mucilaginous texture that is soothing to inflamed tissues in the mouth and throat. It is ideally suited to treat a cough that accompanies a sore throat. Slippery elm cough lozenges have been sold in the United States since the late 1800s. It was an official cough remedy in the United States Pharmacopoeia from 1820 until 1930. It is used to treat coughs in Appalachia today.

Directions: Stir one ounce of slippery elm bark powder and three tablespoons of honey into one pint of boiling water. Let stand, strain, and take one-tablespoon doses as desired.

Mallow

For a dry or inflamed cough high in the respiratory tract that's accompanied by a sore throat, a tea made from marshmallow (*Althea officinalis*) or hollyhock (*Althea rosea*) and honey may bring relief. Both plants have been used in traditional European herbalism at least since the time of the ancient Greeks. The plants came to North America as garden plants and are still used today to treat coughs in professional medical herbalism.

Dried marshmallow root contains up to one-third mucilage. Marshmallow is also expectorant, so the double action of the plant mucilage and its ability to increase natural mucus will help soothe the inflamed membranes of the throat.

Hollyhock flowers may be used instead of marshmallow root. Says the 19th century German herbal *My Water Cure* (English translation), a popular book among German immigrants in the United States, "Among the flowers in the garden, hollyhock must not be missing. When the good creator painted its blossoms, so pleasing to the eye, he poured a drop of medicinal sap into the paint for every petal."

Directions: Cover one ounce of chopped marshmallow root with one pint of boiling water and let steep until cool. Add two tablespoons of honey to a cup of the tea and sip as often as desired. Also, try placing a handful of hollyhock flowers and a handful of dried mullein leaves in a one-pint canning jar. Fill with boiling water, cover, and let stand overnight. Strain, and sweeten with honey. Take ¼-cup doses as desired.

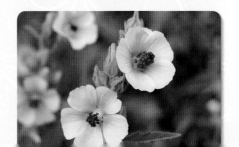

Licorice

Licorice root (*Glycyrrhiza glabra*) has been used to treat coughs and bronchial problems in many traditions throughout the world. It is listed in several 19th century medicinal remedy collections from the eastern United States. It was an official medicine in the United States Pharmacopoeia from 1820 until 1975; it was recommended as a flavoring agent and a demulcent and expectorant for cough syrups. (Most licorice candy in the United States is really flavored with anise oil.)

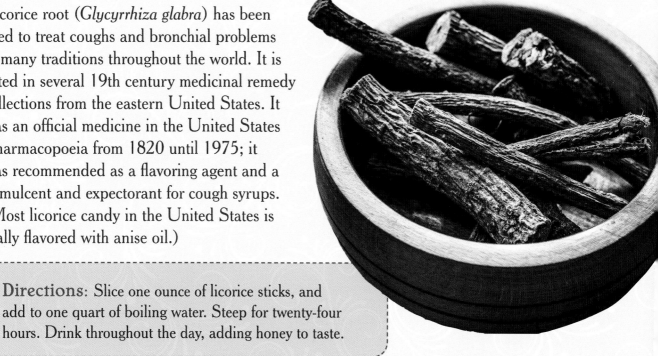

Directions: Slice one ounce of licorice sticks, and add to one quart of boiling water. Steep for twenty-four hours. Drink throughout the day, adding honey to taste.

Ginger

Several North American Indian tribes, including the Allegheny and Montagnais, used wild North American ginger (*Asarum canadensis*) for treating coughs. Cultivated ginger (*Zingiber officinale*) is mentioned for the same purpose in a collection of American remedies called *American Folk Medicine* by folklorist Clarence Meyer. Ginger is commonly used today in Chinese medicine. Ginger contains both anti-inflammatory and antispasmodic chemical constituents.

Directions: Thinly slice a fresh ginger root (about the size of your thumb). Place in one quart of water. Bring to a boil and then simmer in a covered pot on the lowest possible heat for thirty minutes. Let cool for thirty minutes more. Strain and drink a half to one cup, sweetened with honey, as often as desired. Ginger can be irritating to hot, dry, unproductive coughs and should thus be avoided when such a cough is present.

Depression

If you suffer from sadness that is intense and severe, it may not simply be the blues. You could be suffering from depression.

Depression is a psychological condition characterized by prolonged sadness, combined with other symptoms, including persistent low, anxious, or "empty" feelings, decreased energy, loss of interest or pleasure in usual activities, sleep disturbances, and feelings of hopelessness. Depression may be due to an imbalance or lack of certain necessary brain chemicals.

Some types of depression run in families, indicating that a biological vulnerability to the condition can be inherited. Psychological makeup also plays a role in vulnerability to depression. People who have low self-esteem, who consistently view themselves and the world with pessimism, or who are readily overwhelmed by stress are prone to depression. A serious loss, chronic illness, difficult relationship, financial problem, or unwelcome change in life patterns can also trigger a depressive episode.

Depression can occur because of normal chemical changes in the body. Two examples are premenstrual depression and postpartum depression, both thought to be linked to female hormonal activities. In addition, certain drugs, including oral contraceptives, alcohol, and some sedatives, may cause a side effect of depression in some people. Certain infections (including influenza) can depress a person's mood, as can over- or underproduction of hormones by the outer layer of the adrenal gland, or a deficiency of vitamin B12. Scientific evidence has also linked some forms of depression to deficiencies of the vitamins biotin, folic acid, pantothenic acid, pyridoxine, riboflavin, thiamine, vitamin C, and vitamin E. Deficiencies in the minerals calcium, copper, iron, magnesium, potassium, and zinc can also cause depression. (In fact, deficiencies of magnesium and zinc alone can cause symptoms that can lead to a diagnosis of depression. According to the U.S. Department of Agriculture, the average American does not consume the minimum daily requirement of either mineral.) So, before taking antidepressant drugs, patients with mild depression would be wise to undergo a thorough screening of their nutritional status.

Traditional societies are less likely than we are to report depression in their literature because they are more likely to consume a whole-food, nutrient-dense diet and to get sufficient exercise. Weston Price, a nutritional anthropologist who studied traditional societies around the world in the 1930s, found that primitive people consuming a traditional diet take in from three to ten times the vitamin and mineral content found in modern diets.

Very few remedies appear for depression in folk literature; the word itself is a 20th century medical term. Older texts are more likely to refer to depression as melancholy (depressive mood), neurasthenia (nervous exhaustion), malaise (profound fatigue), possession, or witchcraft.

Depression can be very serious. Depression with thoughts of suicide requires immediate medical attention. Conventional treatment for depression includes taking an antidepressant and, sometimes, participating in psychotherapy.

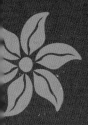
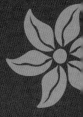

Remedies for *Depression*

St. John's Wort

St. John's wort is a common meadowland plant that has been used as a medicine for centuries. (It is mentioned in early European and Slavic herbals.) The genus name *Hypericum* is from the Latin *hyper*, meaning "above," and *icon*, meaning "spirit." The herb was hung over doorways to ward off evil spirits or burned to protect and sanctify an area. German immigrants to the United States at the turn of the century used it as a digestive herb for "melancholy."

St. John's wort is reported to relieve anxiety and tension and to act as an antidepressant. The herb is an approved medicine in Germany. With long-term use, hypericin, one of the constituents, may make the skin of a few individuals more sensitive to sunlight, however.

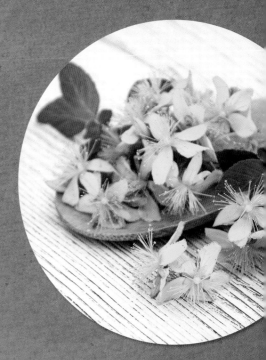

Directions: Purchase St. John's wort from a health food store, herb shop, or pharmacy. Take as directed. Alternately, you can purchase a St. John's wort tincture at a health food store or herb shop. A good quality tincture will be dark red in color.

For a more traditional formula, try this Romani "soul-refreshing tonic":

Gather properly identified wild St. John's wort leaves and flowers, enough to fill a loosely packed pint or quart jar. To follow ancient traditions, harvest them on St. John's day, the day after the summer solstice. (You can do this in most parts of the country, but at higher elevations the flowers will not yet be in bloom, so you'll have to wait a little longer to try this remedy.) Cover the leaves and flowers with ninety proof liquor. Let stand for one cycle of the moon, shaking the bottle daily. Strain and rebottle. Take ten to twenty drops daily.

California Poppy

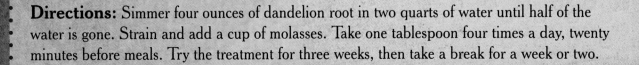

California poppy (*Eschscholtzia californica*) was used as a treatment of the nervous system by the Costanoan Indians. California poppy eventually made its way into European medicine, and today pharmaceutical preparations of the herb are prescribed by physicians in Germany for nervous disorders, including mild depression. The Germans consider the herb to be so gentle that it is sometimes prescribed for treating mild emotional disorders in children. (Although it bears the name "poppy," the herb is not a narcotic and contains no morphine or codeine-type alkaloids.)

California poppy is not readily available in the herb trade, but it grows freely in the western United States and is a common garden plant in other areas. Do not use during pregnancy or while nursing.

Directions: Pick some California poppies, using the stems, leaves, and flowers of the plant. Let them dry in a warm place, out of direct sunlight. Place one teaspoon of the dried herb in a cup and fill the cup with boiling water. Cover and let steep for twenty minutes. Strain and drink one to three cups a day, as desired.

Dandelion

A traditional treatment for "bilious" depression, according to folklorist Clarence Meyer in his book *American Folk Medicine*, combines dandelion root with molasses. This "double-duty" treatment may help depression associated with a sluggish liver while, at the same time, restore mineral deficiencies that contribute to fatigue and low energy. Blackstrap molasses contains high amounts of essential minerals—a tablespoon contains more than fifteen percent of the daily requirement of calcium, magnesium, iron, potassium, copper, and manganese.

Directions: Simmer four ounces of dandelion root in two quarts of water until half of the water is gone. Strain and add a cup of molasses. Take one tablespoon four times a day, twenty minutes before meals. Try the treatment for three weeks, then take a break for a week or two.

Wormwood

Wormwood (*Artemisia absinthum*) has been widely used to treat "melancholy" in European medicine. Also, at least seven North American Indian tribes used it as "witchcraft medicine"—the symptoms of possession and depression may have been similarly interpreted.

In addition to its mild antidepressant effects, wormwood increases the secretion of bile in the liver and has anti-inflammatory properties. Wormwood may be toxic, however, if taken for continually for long periods of time.

Directions: Purchase a wormwood tincture at a health food store or herb shop. Using a dropper, take fifteen drops of the tincture two or three times a day for two to three weeks.

Oats

Oats (*Avena sativa*) are a remedy for neurasthenia, or "nervous exhaustion," which is an old term for the condition. At the turn of the century, the use of oats to treat nervous exhaustion was widespread among the Eclectic physicians, a school of physicians who used herbal remedies.

Oats are highly nutritious. In fact, one cup of oats contains 26 grams of protein, 4 grams of essential fatty acids, 7.4 milligrams of iron, 276 milligrams of magnesium, 0.5 milligrams of copper, 6 milligrams of zinc, 7.1 milligrams of manganese, and 97 micrograms of folic acid—values that are more than half the recommended dietary allowance for each of these nutrients. Clinical research has demonstrated that oats may also aid in withdrawal from addictions.

Directions: Place one cup of oats in three cups of water and simmer for forty minutes in a covered pot. Add molasses or honey to taste. Pour off the liquid and save—you can drink it during the day. Eat the remaining gruel.

DIARRHEA

Whether it's the flu or something you ate, if you're like the average American, you'll suffer once or twice this year from diarrhea.

Diarrhea is abnormally frequent and excessively liquid bowel movements. This is often the body's defensive attempt to rid itself of irritating or toxic substances. It is a symptom that accompanies many disorders, both mild and serious.

There are two basic types of diarrhea: acute (or short-term) diarrhea, the more common form, which comes on quickly and usually lasts no more than two or three days, although it can last as long as two weeks; and chronic (or long-term) diarrhea, which may also appear suddenly but lingers for many weeks or months, with symptoms either constantly present or appearing and disappearing.

Both acute and chronic diarrhea can become a serious problem because of the excessive loss of body fluids (called dehydration) and the loss of the nutrients sodium, potassium, and chloride. Simply drinking more water is not sufficient to replace these losses. Minerals as well as glucose must be replaced in severe di-

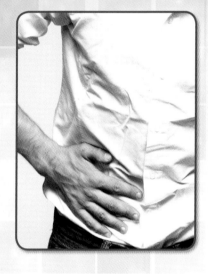

arrhea. Electrolyte replacement drinks for infants are readily available in grocery stores. Use of such replacement liquids has revolutionized diarrhea care for infants throughout the Third World in the last ten years, where diarrhea is a leading cause of infant death. The accompanying sidebar shows the composition of electrolyte replacement formulas.

In an infection, the intestines may pour out massive quantities of fluids and salts in response to a bacterial toxin (poison) or other irritant. Viruses may cause minor epidemics of diarrhea, usually referred to as "intestinal flu." (The influenza virus is actually not

114

involved.) In inflammatory bowel disease (also known as colitis), protein, blood, and mucus are lost through the inflamed lining of the colon; large quantities of water are also lost. Other disorders speed up the normal movement of the colon, thereby not allowing time for absorption of fluids. Yet another type of diarrhea is caused by poor absorption of a type of sugar (called lactose) that draws fluid out of the colon. Other causes of diarrhea include changes in the diet, certain medications, stress, and food allergies. Diarrhea is a symptom and not a disease, and conventional treatment for diarrhea varies widely depending on the cause. Most important is the replacement of fluids and electrolytes if diarrhea is severe. Constipating drugs or bulk fiber may also be given. Common medical wisdom, both conventional and alternative, is to let normal mild diarrhea run its course because it is a natural defense mechanism that washes infectious bacteria, viruses, or toxins out of the body. Diarrhea may be suppressed with constipating astringents, whether herbal or over-the-counter, but that may make you sicker. According to *My Water Cure*, by Father Sebastian Kneipp, a 19th-century German peasant priest and folk healer: "Sudden stopping of diarrhea is never to be recommended: the foul matters should be gradually removed...."

The natural remedies below focus on correcting the cause of the condition.

ELECTROLYTE REPLACEMENT THERAPY

The World Health Organization recommends the following formula for electrolyte replacement after excessive diarrhea or vomiting:

Three and a half grams table salt (sodium chloride)

Two and a half grams baking soda (sodium bicarbonate)

One and a half grams potassium chloride

Twenty grams of glucose

Add the ingredients to a liter (one quart, two ounces) of water and drink.

For electrolyte replacement, you can also try the formula below. This remedy, taken from a German medical text, includes peppermint, which is a traditional treatment for diarrhea.

Directions: Make a tea by simmering one tablespoon each of peppermint leaves and fennel seed in one covered quart of water for fifteen minutes. Strain and allow to cool to room temperature. Add ½ teaspoon salt, ¼ teaspoon baking soda, ¼ teaspoon potassium chloride, and two tablespoons glucose. Drink freely.

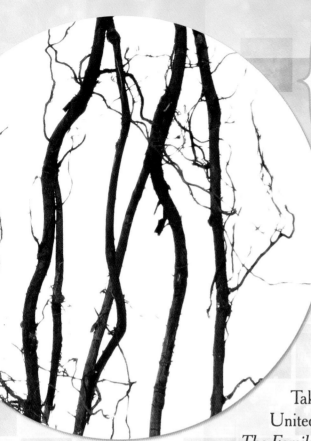

Remedies for
DIARRHEA

Blackberry Root

Perhaps the most commonly recommended remedy for diarrhea in North American literature is blackberry root tea. Blackberry roots (*Rubus hispidus*) are not usually available in the commercial herb trade, but, if you are willing to brave the thorns, then start picking—the plant grows throughout most of the United States.

Taking blackberry root was a popular remedy in the United States during the 1800s. A listing in the 1849 book *The Family Physician* states that blackberry root "often provides a sovereign remedy [for diarrhea] when all other remedies fail." The text states that, during a dysentery epidemic, none of the local Indians using blackberry root died, while many of their white neighbors did. The root was used to treat diarrhea by the Oneida, Rappahannock, and Shinnecock Indians. It was likely that the whites died of mercury poisoning—mercury was what the white physicians used to treat diarrhea at the time.

The use of blackberry root for treating diarrhea survives today in the natural medicine of New England, Indiana, Appalachia, and among the Amish in the eastern states. The roots contain astringent tannins, which dry up the watery secretions of the intestines. The following suggestion comes from the traditions of New England.

DIRECTIONS: Simmer a handful of the roots in one pint of water until the liquid turns dark. Drink one cup. Wait a few hours and, if necessary, drink another. Don't take more than two cups a day. Gather the roots in the fall.

Wormwood

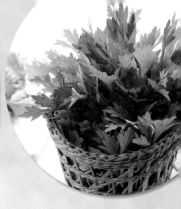

German immigrants at the turn of the century used wormwood tincture (*Artemisia absinthium*) to treat diarrhea. They arrived in this country carrying with them a popular health book called *My Water Cure* (English translation) by Father Sebastian Kneipp. The book warned against taking the remedy for a prolonged period of time or at high doses.

In the past, Europeans who consumed large amounts of wormwood, via an alcoholic drink called "absinthe," developed a form of insanity. The artist Vincent Van Gogh probably suffered from this mental illness, which may account for his progressive insanity and the increasing hallucinatory quality of his paintings at the end of his life.

DIRECTIONS: Purchase a tincture of wormwood in a health food store. Take a dropperful three times a day for no more than two days for treating simple diarrhea.

Charcoal

The use of charcoal for treating diarrhea in North America was well under way before the arrival of the European colonists. The Kwakiutl tribe from the Pacific Northwest would burn the bark of a fir tree, pulverize the coals, add the ash to water (sometimes with other herbs), and drink the mixture to end diarrhea. The use of "hardwood ashes" in water to treat diarrhea is also recorded by folklorist Clarence Meyer in his folk collection *American Folk Medicine*. Today, the use of charcoal to treat diarrhea is used by the Amish and Seventh Day Adventists.

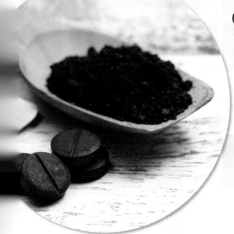

Charcoal is absorbent, meaning that toxic substances attach to it and are tightly bound. It is used in emergency medicine to treat some types of poisoning. Be sure to use activated charcoal, which is very finely powdered and treated to be free of contaminants and gases.

DIRECTIONS: Purchase charcoal capsules from a pharmacy. Take four to eight capsules three to four times a day.

Diarrhea

Orange Peel

In reference to orange peel, a 9th-century medical text from Baghdad, Iraq, says that "candied skin" is good for the stomach. Orange peel teas were used to treat digestive problems in Arabic medicine and European medicine during the Middle Ages, until the 1600s. The peels of related citrus fruits are still used for treating digestive complaints in China and India today. The practice also survives in the traditions of Indiana.

The oils in the peels stimulate digestion. (Today, dyes and pesticides are used on oranges, so if you want to try this remedy, you'll have to obtain organic oranges.) An Indiana remedy says to drink freely of orange peel tea sweetened with sugar.

DIRECTIONS: Peel one organic orange and chop the skin into small pieces. Place the skin in a pot and cover with one pint of boiling water. Cover well and let stand until the water reaches room temperature. Sweeten with sugar or honey and drink freely.

Chamomile (German)

German immigrants to the United States used German chamomile (*Matricaria recutita*) to treat diarrhea. Chamomile is also mentioned as a treatment for diarrhea in Romani folklore.

Chamomile contains strong anti-inflammatory oils as well as other active principles. It may be best used in treating diarrhea caused by intestinal inflammation. Modern studies show it has antispasmodic properties as well. One German source suggests combining the tea half-and-half with peppermint. A Romani treatment calls for adding twenty-five blueberries to the tea. Thus, chamomile is probably viewed in natural medicine as a supportive treatment rather than a singular one. The following suggestion offers contemporary German advice.

DIRECTIONS: Add one teaspoon of chamomile flowers and one teaspoon of peppermint leaves in a cup. Add boiling water. Cover and steep for fifteen minutes. Drink three cups a day.

DIGESTION

According to traditional medical systems of Greece, India, and China, the digestive tract is the root of the tree of good health.

If the digestive tract is healthy and digestion and absorption of the nutrients are efficient, then the entire body will be well-nourished and will function optimally. Any irregularity in digestion, however, can cause or contribute to disease anywhere in the body.

Below are some common signs of a poorly functioning digestive system:

- flatulence or belching
- nausea
- pain anywhere in the digestive tract
- undigested food in the stool
- offensive breath
- constipation (less than one bowel movement per day)
- lethargy or depression after meals
- food cravings other than normal hunger
- lack of satisfaction after meals
- lack of hunger for breakfast

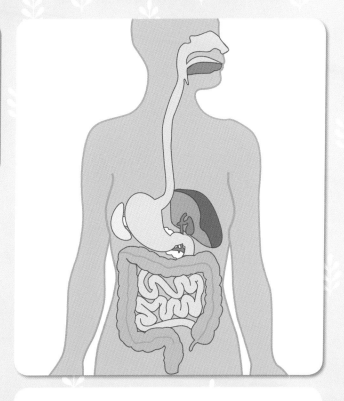

These symptoms—all considered to be serious signs that require treatment in traditional medical systems—are often left untreated by conventional physicians in North America. This is not so in the modern medicine of Germany and France, however, where symptoms such as "biliousness" (sluggish liver function), poor appetite, gas, and bloating, or feelings of fullness after meals, are routinely treated by doctors, often with herbal medicines from the European tradition.

Digestion

According to natural medicine throughout the world, which offers many remedies for weak and sluggish digestion, healthy digestion requires:

- A balance of fats, proteins, and starches in the diet, and adequate fiber from sources such as grains, beans, fruits, and vegetables.

- A moderate intake of food quantities. Overeating strains the capacity of the digestive system to process the consumed food, and undigested or partially digested remnants can cause inflammation and other problems in the digestive tract and elsewhere in the body.

- A relaxed state during meals. For the stomach and intestines to function normally, and for digestive secretions to be adequate, the body cannot be in a state of stress during meals.

- A healthy number of normal bacteria in the gut.

The "garden" of friendly bacteria in the intestines acts as a defense against harmful bacteria, yeasts, molds, and other micro-organisms by competing with them for food. (As the friendly bacteria proliferate, the nutrients they consume deprive the harmful microorganisms of their food supply.) Some of these friendly bacteria manufacture essential vitamins. The good bacteria can be disrupted by courses of such drugs as birth control pills, steroids, and antibiotics, however, leading to poor digestion and inflammation and infection of the intestinal wall. This in turn can cause inflammatory diseases in other parts of the body as the intestinal contents leak through the inflamed gut wall and overwhelm the immune system.

Natural remedies may improve digestion by stimulating the secretion of more stomach acid, digestive enzymes, and bile (a digestive secretion of the liver) from the liver. The remedies may also improve the absorption of nutrients by increasing blood flow to the mucous membranes of the intestines. Finally, antispasmodic constituents in some remedies may prevent spasms in intestinal wall muscles that often accompanies gas and bloating.

Any severe or persistent digestive tract symptoms merit a visit to your doctor.

Bitter Tonics

In natural medicine and traditional herbalism, bitter tonics are one of the most often prescribed categories of herbs and foods. In fact, a 1994 poll of the most-often prescribed medicinal herbs by North American professional herbalists showed that half of the top ten herbs had important bitter constituents.

The key indication for bitter tonics is poor appetite. The bitter constituents in the plants stimulate the secretion of stomach acid and liver bile, thereby improving digestion and nourishment. Because they stimulate these secretions, however, they are contraindicated if you have heartburn or other kinds of digestive pain.

Bitter tonics in this section include wormwood, chamomile, goldenseal, Oregon grape root, gentian, and boneset. Bitter tonics are often combined with carminative herbs in simple formulas.

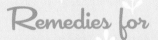

Remedies for
DIGESTION PROBLEMS

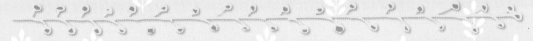

Ginger

Ginger (*Zingiber officinale*) is a remedy for treating gas or nausea in the traditions of both New England and the southern Appalachians. It is used the same way in the traditional medicine of India, China, and Arabia. Ginger contains at least thirteen antispasmodic constituents, which may help reduce spasms and tension in the digestive tract muscles. Also, circulatory stimulants in ginger increase circulation to the mucous membrane lining of the digestive tract, which in turn increases digestive secretions and absorption of nutrients. What's more, in clinical trials, ginger has shown to be effective in soothing some kinds of nausea and vertigo. Avoid excessive doses of ginger if you're taking drugs for heart or blood conditions or diabetes.

Directions: Stir ½ teaspoon of ground ginger into a cup of hot water. Let stand two to three minutes. Strain and drink.

Mint

Different types of mints are recommended for treating indigestion in North American literature, most commonly peppermint (*Mentha piperita*) and spearmint (*Mentha spicata*). Mints appear in the medicine of New England, New York, Indiana, Appalachia, New Mexico, and California. Mints have also been used as carminatives by members of the Cherokee, Chippewa, Dakota, Omaha, Pawnee, Ponca, and Winnebago American Indian tribes. Mint species contain the antispasmodic constituents carvacrol, eugenol, limonene, and thymol, which may help reduce intestinal spasms. A contemporary German medical text, *Herbal Medicine* by R.F. Weiss, M.D., recommends the mints as digestive aids for their carminative and antispasmodic properties. Peppermint is used as an official digestive aid in Germany.

Directions: Place one teaspoon of the dried herb in a cup and add boiling water. Cover and let stand for ten minutes. Strain well and drink the tea warm three times a day on an empty stomach. Don't use peppermint if you are experiencing heartburn or painful belches.

Fennel

A tea of fennel seeds (*Foeniculum vulgare*) is used for treating sluggish digestion or gas in the medicine of both New England and China. It is also the most often prescribed tea for abdominal cramping and gas in adults in the medical herbalism of contemporary Great Britain, Canada, and the United States. It is an approved medicine in Germany for mild gastrointestinal complaints. At least sixteen chemical constituents in fennel have demonstrated antispasmodic effects in animal trials.

Directions: Place one teaspoon of the seeds in a cup and add boiling water. Cover and let stand for ten minutes. Strain and drink three cups of warm tea a day on an empty stomach until digestion improves.

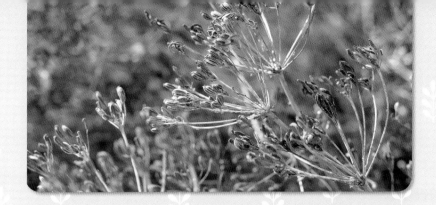

Caraway Seeds

Caraway seeds (*Carum carvi*), with a flavor and a medicinal action similar to that of fennel, are recommended for gas and poor digestion in Appalachia and in the medicine of Indiana. Their medicinal use originated in Arab culture. Their use for poor digestion spread to ancient Rome, and from there to European medicine. Caraway seeds are approved for medical use for weak digestion by the German government.

Directions: In a cup, pour boiling water over one teaspoon of the crushed seeds. Cover and let stand for ten minutes. Strain well and drink three cups of warm tea a day on an empty stomach.

Alternately, you can chew on the seeds. A common practice in households in India and the Middle East is to pass a small bowl of caraway, fennel, or anise seeds for nibbling after meals.

Chamomile (German)

Chamomile (*Matricaria recutita*) is recommended for intestinal spasm or gas in the traditions of New England, Indiana, and the American Southwest. It combines both antispasmodic and sedative properties and may relieve intestinal cramping and induce relaxation at the same time. Chamomile contains at least nineteen antispasmodic constituents, as well as five sedative ones. The plant is approved in Germany as a medicine for gastrointestinal complaints. Also, a 1993 clinical trial in Germany showed that chamomile was effective in relieving infant colic.

Directions: Pour boiling water over one tablespoon of chamomile flowers in a cup. Cover and let sit for ten minutes. Strain and drink warm three times a day on an empty stomach. Do this for two to three weeks. Taking one of the doses before bed may also work as a sleep aid. Avoid using if signs of allergy appear. Avoid excessive use during pregnancy and lactation.

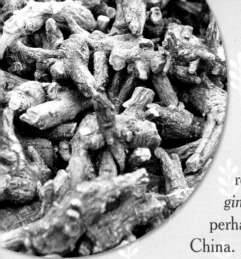

American Ginseng

American ginseng (*Panax quinquefolium*) is used as a digestive tonic throughout the Appalachian mountain chain where it grows. A related species of ginseng (*Panax ginseng*), known as Asian ginseng, is perhaps the most famous tonic herb in China. (American ginseng, however, is also exported to China in large quantities.)

Even though both species are called "ginseng," the Chinese use the two plants for entirely different purposes. Asian ginseng is considered to be stimulating; in fact, it is sometimes used in large doses as a stimulant in Chinese hospital emergency rooms. American ginseng, however, is used as a sedative for individuals who are tense and nervous from prolonged stress or illness.

American ginseng earned the attention of the turn-of-the-20th-century medical doctor Arthur Harding, M.D., who, out of disillusionment with the conventional medicines of his day, abandoned his regular medical practice in order to investigate natural remedies. He said in his book *Ginseng and Other Medicinal Plants*, published in 1909: "If the people of the United States were educated as to its use, our supply of ginseng would be consumed in our own country and it would be a hard blow to the medical profession." In his book, Harding recounts case studies of patients whose generally deteriorated health improved only after a few weeks or months of treatment with ginseng. He attributes the plant's power to restore health to its ability to restore digestion.

Unlike Asian ginseng, very little scientific research has been performed on American ginseng. Thus, we have to rely on contemporary Chinese medicine or on the natural traditions of this country for guidance on its use.

Directions:
American ginseng can cost more than $200 a pound, and many adulterated or ineffective products are sold in health food stores. The most reliable way to use it is to make your own powder from whole roots with the fine rootlets attached.

Purchase the roots and grind them into powder in a coffee grinder. (Consume the powder from one root before grinding another, because the constituents are more likely to be preserved in the whole root than in the powder.) Stir ¼ to ½ teaspoon of the powder into one cup of warm water and drink one dose daily on any empty stomach before breakfast for two to three weeks. Then, repeat if desired after taking a break for one or two weeks.

Wormwood

Wormwood (*Artemisia absinthium, Artemisia* spp.) is described as a digestive stimulant in the Hispanic medicine of southern California. The active constituents of wormwood include bitter digestive stimulants and anti-inflammatory volatile oils including azulenes, constituents that are also present in chamomile. The European species of the plant is approved as a digestive stimulant by the German government.

Directions: Place one teaspoon of wormwood leaves in a cup of water and fill with boiling water. Cover well to prevent the escape of aromatic substances. Let cool to room temperature. Take ½ doses three or four times a day. Don't take wormwood for more than ten days at a time and take a ten-day break before starting the therapy again. Avoid excessive consumption.

Cinnamon

Cinnamon (*Cinnamomum verum*) is used as a digestive stimulant in the medicine of New England and China. It is also used for this purpose in the Hispanic medicine of the Southwest. Cinnamon contains at least sixteen different antispasmodic constituents, especially in its aromatic oils. It contains the antispasmodic and circulatory stimulant cinnamaldehyde in large quantities. Cinnamon is approved by the German government for treatment of poor digestion. It is contraindicated in medicinal quantities during pregnancy, however, because it can stimulate uterine contractions.

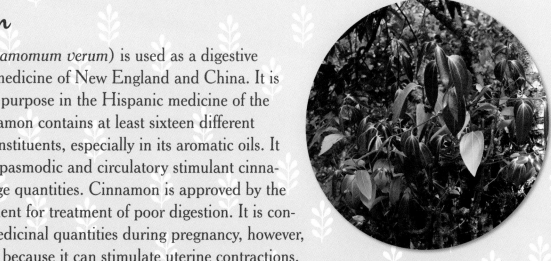

Directions: Stir ¼ to ½ teaspoon of cinnamon powder into a cup of hot water. Let stand three to five minutes. Stir again and drink without straining.

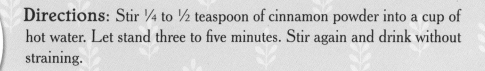

Digestion

Gentian

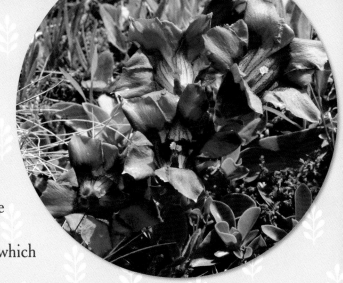

In this country, five of the six North American gentian species were used as digestive aids or bitter tonics by American Indians. Gentian (*Gentiana lutea*) is the most famous component of the pre-dinner "bitters" commonly consumed in European natural medicine. (Bitters are traditionally taken in many cultures ten to twenty minutes before meals to improve the appetite.) Experiments show that bitters increase the secretion of stomach acid, which helps the digestive system prepare for the meal.

The use of gentian also appears in the contemporary literature of British Columbia. Gentian is approved as a bitter tonic by the German government. Like other strong bitters, it is contraindicated if you are experiencing heartburn or other digestive pain or if you have an ulcer.

Directions: Chop up three fresh lemon peels and place with one ounce of chopped gentian root in one quart of water. Bring to a boil and simmer on the lowest heat for ten minutes. Let stand until the tea reaches room temperature. Strain and store in the refrigerator. Take a teaspoon twenty minutes before meals. If the gentian causes heartburn, stop taking it. Avoid in pregnancy and lactation.

Gentian & Ginger

In natural medicine, gentian is usually combined with other herbs or foods to make pre-dinner bitters (see "Gentian," above). Gentian is most commonly combined with a warming, spicy herb.

Directions: Grind some gentian root in a coffee grinder to make a powder. Mix well with an equal amount of powdered ginger root. Stir ¼ to ½ teaspoon of the mixture into a cup of hot water. Let stand three to five minutes. Stir again and drink, without straining, twenty minutes before meals. If this remedy causes heartburn, try a different one.

Goldenseal & Oregon Grape Root

Goldenseal (*Hydrastis canadensis*) is the most famous bitter tonic in North American natural medicine. The colonists learned its use from the American Indians, and it entered into the folk medicine of New England in the 1700s. Goldenseal remained a common household remedy throughout the eastern states during the 1800s. It was also one of the most commonly prescribed herbs by doctors of the Eclectic and Physiomedicalist schools of medicine.

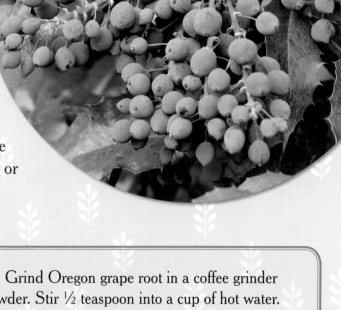

Although goldenseal had several therapeutic uses, the physicians often prescribed it to restore the functioning of a "run-down" digestive system.

In the modern day, goldenseal is an endangered species, so medical herbalists in North America frequently prescribe Oregon grape root (*Mahonia aquifolium, Berberis aquifolium*) as a substitute bitter tonic. (Because of its equivalent bitter effects, Eclectic physicians also prescribed Oregon grape root.) As with other strong bitters, don't take either of these herbs if you are experiencing digestive pain or if you have an ulcer.

Directions: Grind Oregon grape root in a coffee grinder to make a powder. Stir ½ teaspoon into a cup of hot water. Allow to stand for three to five minutes. Don't strain, just stir. Drink the cup twenty minutes before meals for one to three weeks.

Boneset

Contemporary North Carolina traditions suggest taking a tea of boneset (*Eupatorium perfoliatum*) for weak digestion. Boneset was one of the most common natural remedies in the early American colonies, where it was considered to be a panacea (a cure all). It was taken as a hot tea to treat colds, flu, and feverish diseases. As a cold tea, it was used as a bitter digestive tonic. Boneset is very bitter to the taste.

Directions: Place one tablespoon of dried boneset leaves in a one-pint jar and fill with boiling water. Cover and let cool to room temperature. Drink half of a cup twenty minutes before meals for one to three weeks.

Thyme

A digestive stimulant found in the traditions of both Indiana and China is thyme (*Thymus vulgaris*). Thymol, the chief aromatic substance of thyme that gives it its fragrance, has antispasmodic and carminative properties. Animal research has shown that thymol relaxes the muscles of the intestinal tract, which relieves pressure from gas.

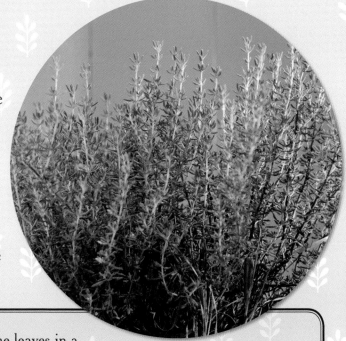

Directions: Place one teaspoon of dried thyme leaves in a cup and fill with boiling water. Let stand, covered, for ten minutes. Strain and drink. Do this three times a day, before meals, on an empty stomach. Thyme oil is toxic and should only be used when highly diluted.

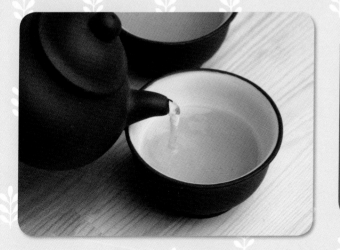

Catnip

Catnip (*Nepeta cataria*) tea, a sedative and indigestion remedy in European natural medicine, has been a popular remedy in this country since the arrival of the European immigrants. The plant rapidly became naturalized here, and American Indian tribes such as the Onondaga and Cayuga eventually used it for poor digestion as well, especially when treating children. It was an official medicine in the United States Pharmacopoeia from 1840 until 1870.

Catnip has been used in natural medicine to treat weak digestion, intestinal spasm, and gas by residents of New England, Appalachia, North Carolina, Indiana, and New Mexico and by Blacks throughout the deep South and by Chicanos in Los Angeles. Catnip combines both carminative and sedative properties, with seven antispasmodic and five sedative constituents.

Directions: Pour boiling water over one teaspoon of the dried herb. Let sit covered for ten minutes. Strain and drink three cups a day, between meals on an empty stomach.

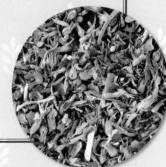

ECZEMA

The cause of eczema is unknown, although allergies may play a role in triggering outbreaks. Find relief with a remedy below.

Eczema is an inflammation of the skin and is most commonly equated with the medical term atopic dermatitis. It is characterized by red, oozing, and sometimes crusty lesions on the face, the scalp, the extremities, and the diaper area in infants. The lesions may also become infected with bacteria or other microorganisms, and infection with herpes virus can cause serious illness. Stress, food allergens, scratching, bathing, and sweating may also induce attacks.

Conventional treatment includes avoidance of triggers and administration of antihistamine topical steroid creams and antibiotics for infections of the eczema lesions. Alternative medical treatments include avoidance of triggers; optimizing vitamin, mineral, and essential fatty acid nutrition to reduce tendency to develop inflammation; internal or topical applications of anti-inflammatory or soothing herbs; and administration of bitter herbs to "stimulate the liver" and optimize digestion.

In alternative medicine, it is believed that to heal the skin, you must heal the digestive tract as well. Thus, a three-way link that exists between the liver, the digestive tract, and the skin is a key tenet of alternative medicine for treating allergic eczema and other skin inflammations. One physiological basis for this theory may be the detoxifying role of the liver. The liver normally transforms toxic substances so they can be excreted from the body either in the form of bile from the liver or as urine. If the liver is not doing its job, toxic substances may circulate freely in the body and irritate the skin "from the inside out."

The natural treatments in this section include bitter herbs to stimulate the liver and digestive tract, anti-inflammatory herbs for both internal and external use, astringent and disinfectant herbs for topical use, and treatments with water and clay.

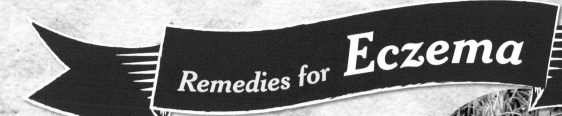

Nettle & Dandelion

A Romani remedy for eczema uses a combination of two "blood purifying" herbs that are traditionally prescribed to treat skin conditions. Stinging nettle (*Urtica dioica, U. urens*) has been used by at least seven American Indian tribes—from the northeastern United States to the Pacific Northwest and down to Mexico—as an aid for healing skin conditions. Stinging nettle is used for the same purpose in traditional European herbalism. A recent clinical trial showed that nettle was effective for treating hay fever, and recent laboratory research has identified its anti-inflammatory and anti-allergic constituents.

Dandelion root is traditionally considered to be a "liver" herb —its use in this country is consistent with the traditional idea of treating skin ailments through the liver (see introduction to this section, opposite page). It has been used to treat skin conditions by several American Indian tribes, including the Iroquois of the northeastern United States, the Aleuts of the Pacific Northwest, and the Tewa of the Southwest. The German government has approved the medicinal use of dandelion root as a "cholagogue," a medicine that increases the flow of bile from the liver. Constituents in dandelion have also been found to protect the liver and to enhance its detoxifying ability. Dandelion contains both antioxidant and anti-inflammatory constituents.

Directions: Place one ounce of dandelion root and one ounce of nettle leaf in a pot, and cover with three pints of water. Boil and then simmer, covered, on low heat for forty minutes. Cool to room temperature. Drink three cups a day. Do this for three weeks, and then take a break for seven to ten days before starting again.

Burdock Root

In the traditional herbalism of Europe and North America, burdock (*Arctium lappa, A. minus*) is probably the most well-known for treating skin complaints such as acne, boils, or eczema. It has been used to treat skin conditions by several American Indian tribes, including the Cherokee, Iroquois, Menominee, Micmac, Nanticoke, and Penobscot. Burdock is used today in natural medicine as a "blood purifier" among Pennsylvania Germans, the Amish, Indiana farmers, and throughout Appalachia. Burdock was an official medicine in the United States Pharmacopoeia from 1831 until 1842, and again from 1851 until 1916; it was prescribed as a diuretic, mild laxative, and treatment for skin ailments.

Modern scientific studies show that constituents in burdock root have anti-inflammatory properties. Its constituent poly-saccharide inulin, which can make up fifty percent of the root by weight, provides food for the "friendly" strains of bacteria in the gut and may thus help reduce the toxic load on the liver and skin by reducing toxicity in the bowels.

For some individuals, however, burdock can worsen eczema. Perhaps this is because burdock promotes light sweating, and sweat can trigger eczema in some people. If you find that burdock makes your eczema worse, stop using it immediately and try a different remedy.

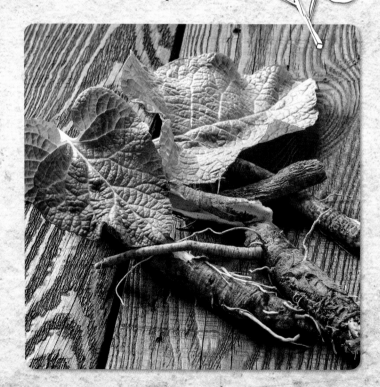

Directions: Put one ounce of burdock root in one quart of water. Bring to a boil and simmer, covered, for forty minutes. Drink the quart throughout the day. Burdock is a mild herb and can be consumed this way for long periods of time.

Yellow Dock

Yellow dock (*Rumex crispus*), like dandelion and burdock, is a traditional bitter, liver-stimulating herb. The Aleut, Cherokee, Cheyenne, Iroquois, Navaho, and Shoshone Indians, as well as other American Indian tribes, used it to treat skin ailments. It was a remedy for treating eczema of residents of the eastern states in the 1800s. It was listed in the United States Pharmacopoeia from 1860 until 1890; physicians of the last century used it to treat chronic skin ailments. It is still used today for this purpose in the Southwest.

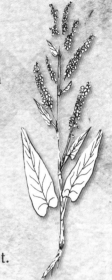

Directions: Make a tincture of yellow dock by placing four ounces of the dried root in a one-quart jar and filling the jar with 100 proof vodka or gin. Let stand for three weeks, shaking the jar once a day. Strain and store in a cool dark place. The dose is two to three droppers twice a day, taken in a cup of warm water. Alternately, you can purchase a tincture of yellow dock at a health food or herb store.

Baking Soda Bath

Contemporary Seventh Day Adventists recommend treating eczema by taking a baking soda bath. In New England, the same treatment is used for relieving hives, itching, rashes, and other skin conditions.

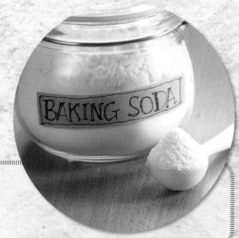

Directions: Place a few handfuls of baking soda in warm bath water and take a long soak.

Eczema

Fringe Tree Bark

A contemporary Appalachian treatment for eczema is taking fringe tree bark (*Chionanthus virginicus*). This bitter, liver-stimulating herb was one of the top ten most-often prescribed herbs by the Eclectic physicians in 1920; they used it to treat liver diseases in particular. American Indians used it externally on cuts, wounds, and skin inflammations. (Use external applications to treat eczema.)

Though fringe tree bark has been studied very little by modern scientists, its reputation persists thanks to its former popularity. Internal use requires a tincture. Use as a tea when applying as an external wash.

Directions: Purchase a tincture of fringe tree bark at a health food store. Take a dropperful three times a day for seven to ten days. Discontinue if any digestive discomfort develops.

To apply as an external wash, simmer one tablespoon of the bark in a cup of boiling water for fifteen minutes. Strain and, using gauze, apply to the eczema.

Honey

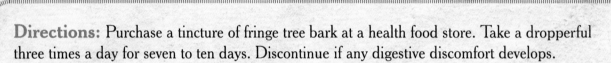

Honey is a traditional remedy for infected eczema throughout Asia. Honey is also used by Chinese Americans. Honey is a powerful disinfectant and has been used by conventional physicians in both France and India as a disinfectant for burns.

Directions: Cover gauze with a layer of honey, place over the eczema, and cover with tape or a bandage. Change the dressing every two hours until the infection is gone.

Oregon Grape Root & Yellow Dock

American Indian tribes in the North Central and Pacific Northwest states took Oregon grape internally to treat the digestive tract and applied it externally to treat skin conditions. The Cowlitz Indians applied it externally as a disinfectant; today, physicians in Germany use it in the same way for treating psoriasis.

The contemporary Amish use a combination of Oregon grape root (*Berberis aquifolium*) and yellow dock root (*Rumex crispus*) for treating eczema. Oregon grape, like yellow dock, is considered in contemporary British and North American herbalism to be a liver herb, and its constituents berberine, berbamine, and oxyacanthine all promote the flow of bile.

Directions: Purchase a tincture of Oregon grape root and some capsules of powdered yellow dock root. Take one dropper of the Oregon grape tincture and four capsules of the yellow dock root three times a day until the eczema is relieved. In addition, dilute one ounce of the Oregon grape tincture with five ounces of water, and apply the diluted solution, using gauze or a clean cloth, to the eczema.

Thyme

Another traditional Chinese remedy for treating eczema is to wash the affected area with a tea of thyme leaves (*Thymus vulgaris*). Thyme leaves contain about two percent thymol, a volatile constituent that has strong antiseptic and anti-inflammatory properties.

Directions: Place one ounce of thyme leaves in a one-quart canning jar and fill with boiling water. Cover tightly to prevent the thymol from escaping with the steam. Let cool to room temperature. Apply to eczema with gauze or a clean cloth three or four times a day. If you find the remedy irritating, dilute it in half and try again.

Eczema

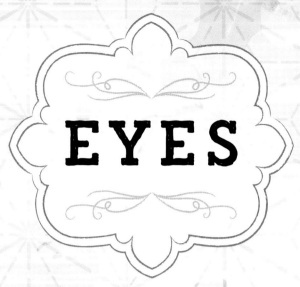

EYES

The most common natural remedies for the eyes help to relieve soreness and infection. Soothe your eyes with one of the remedies below.

Conjunctivitis, or pinkeye, is an inflammation of the conjunctiva. The conjunctiva is a delicate membrane that lines the inner surface of the eyelid and covers the exposed surface of the eye. Most cases of conjunctivitis result from disease-causing microorganisms such as bacteria, fungi, and viruses. Allergies, chemicals, dust, smoke, and foreign objects that irritate the conjunctiva may also lead to conjunctivitis. (Occasionally a sexually transmitted disease can cause pinkeye if the eyes are rubbed after touching infected genital organs. Herpes simplex keratitis is a painful viral infection of the cornea of the eye that can result in blindness if not treated.)

Most cases of conjunctivitis in North America are caused by viruses. In Asia and the Mediterranean region, however, eye infections are commonly caused by the organism *Chlamydia trachomatis*. Known as trachoma, this persistent infection can cause scarring and excessive drying of the membranes around the eyes and lead to blindness.

Conventional treatment depends upon the cause and resulting symptoms of the conjunctivitis. If the inflammation is environmentally caused, simply removing the irritant may be sufficient to eliminate the condition. For more difficult cases, a physician may prescribe antibiotics, steroids, or combination eye drops to be used several times a day as directed.

Pass the Cream

A New England remedy for treating a wide variety of eye problems—including tired, sore, itchy, ulcerated, or infected eyes—is to put a few drops of milk or cream in the eye. In the past, American Indians of the Rappahannock tribe used human breast milk in the same way. Today, contemporary residents of the southern Appalachians use the breast milk method. Human breast milk contains antibodies against many organisms and may help fight a local infection of the eye.

A most important fact about conjunctivitis is that its infectious form is highly contagious. Individuals with infective conjunctivitis should not share handkerchiefs, towels, or washcloths. You should be careful to avoid touching the unaffected eye after touching or rubbing the infected eye because it can easily become infected as well.

The most common natural remedies for the eyes focus on relieving infected, sore, or tired eyes as well as removing irritating objects. (Of course, caution should be used when removing a foreign object from the eye. Sometimes even small objects can tear the surface of the eyeball or cornea, and infection can result. So use common sense, and if the irritation is severe, soreness persists after removal of the object, or infection or inflammation follow the incident, seek prompt medical advice.) The natural treatments for treating conjunctivitis commonly employ drying substances, which give tone to swollen membranes around the eyes. Some of the herbs recommended also have antibacterial, antiviral, and anti-inflammatory properties.

Any persistent eye irritation or infection requires a medical checkup.

Treating Trachoma

Both goldenseal (*Hydrastis canadensis*) and Oregon grape root (*Mahonia aquifolium, Berberis aquifolium*) contain the constituent berberine. Berberine is used in Asia to treat eye infections caused by the organism *Chlamydia trachomatis*, a bacteria that can spread directly from an affected person's eyes or indirectly from flies or contaminated clothing. This infection, called trachoma, is the most common cause of blindness in southern and southeastern Asia. Berberine sulfate was found in one clinical trial to be more effective than the most commonly used pharmaceutical antibiotic for the condition, especially when it is used to prevent recurrences. Berberine sulfate is also used to treat diarrheal infections in Asia.

Neither of the above plants have been tested in clinical trials in this country for their ability to treat trachoma, but both have been used to treat this condition in American natural medicine—goldenseal in the eastern United States where it grows, and Oregon grape root in the western states.

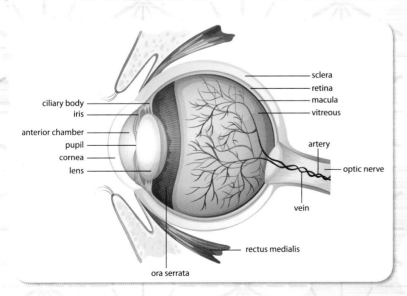

ciliary body
iris
anterior chamber
pupil
cornea
lens
sclera
retina
macula
vitreous
artery
optic nerve
vein
rectus medialis
ora serrata

Remedies for the EYES

ROSE

Today, rose (*Rosa* spp.) is among the most often pre-scribed herbs in Unani Tibb, which is contemporary Arabic medicine. The use of rose as an eyewash may well have come to the American Southwest by way of the Arabs. The Arabs, who controlled Spain for the 800 years preceding the Spanish colonization of North America, had a profound effect on Hispanic culture and medicine.

Rose petals have a strong astringent action, toning up swollen and inflamed mucous membranes. This is their chief medicinal use in Arabic medicine.

Hispanics in northern New Mexico use rose petal tea as an eyewash. The rose oil in the leaves contains fifteen bactericidal, nine antiviral, and seven anti-inflammatory constituents.

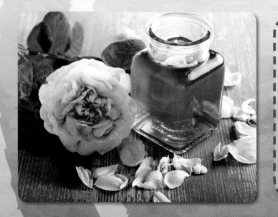

DIRECTIONS: Obtain rose petals from wild or garden-cultivated roses that are free of pesticides and chemicals. (Most commercial roses are sprayed with a variety of chemicals.) Place a handful of petals in a jar and add one pint of boiling water. Cover well to retain the aromatic oils, and let stand until the water reaches room temperature. Apply to the eyes with a clean cloth.

TEA

Tea is used to treat eye conditions in the natural medicine of southern Appalachia; it is used in the natural medicine of India and Asia as well. Tea and tea leaves are used to treat all types

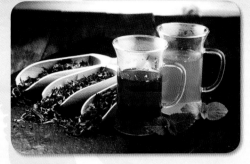

of eyes irritations and infections, including runny eyes, conjunctivitis, particles in the eye, swollen eyelids, sticky eyelids, and eyes red from a hangover.

Tea is a virtual pharmacy of chemical constituents: The leaves contain thirty-four antibacterial substances, sixteen antiviral substances, and twenty-four anti-inflammatory constituents. Tea leaves also have a strong astringent action, which soothes infected membranes.

DIRECTIONS: Make a tea using black or green tea bags or by adding one teaspoon of tea leaves to one cup of boiling water. Apply a tea-soaked cloth or a used tea bag, to the eyes. Keep in place ten to fifteen minutes. Repeat as desired.

WITCH HAZEL

Although eastern American Indians have used witch hazel (*Hamamelis virginiana*) to treat a variety of conditions, the Chippewa Indians used it specifically to treat sore, inflamed, or infected eyes. Modern New England natural medicine continues to use witch hazel in this manner.

Witch hazel is a tree native to North America. After colonists learned its importance from the Indians, its use for healing spread to Europe, where it is still prescribed today in professional British herbalism and in conventional German medicine. The German government, after reviewing scientific evidence, has approved its use for minor inflammations of the skin and mucous membranes. Witch hazel products are available in most drug stores and health food stores.

DIRECTIONS: Purchase witch hazel leaves at a health food store or herb shop. Do not use commercial alcohol-based preparations—the alcohol will irritate your eyes. Place one teaspoon of the leaves in a cup and fill with boiling water. Cover and let stand until the water reaches room temperature. Moisten a cloth in the tea and apply to shut eyes.

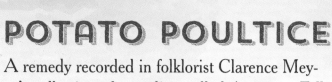

POTATO POULTICE

A remedy recorded in folklorist Clarence Meyer's collection of remedies, called *American Folk Medicine*, is the potato poultice. Presumably, the starch in the potato acts to soothe the inflammation in the eye. Small amounts of a number of other anti-inflammatory constituents are also present in the potato.

The potato is native to the Andes mountains in South America. Its use as a food spread throughout Europe in the 1700s. It is used today in European natural medicine to soothe painful joints, headaches, and other inflammatory conditions.

DIRECTIONS: Remove the skin from a whole, raw potato. Wash the potato and dry well. Grate as fine as possible. Place inside a clean cloth and fold to make a poultice. Place the poultice over the inflamed eye for fifteen minutes.

OREGON GRAPE ROOT

A tea of the roots or leaves of Oregon grape root (*Mahonia* spp., *Berberis aquifolium*) was used as an eyewash by American Indians of both the mountainous American Southwest and the Pacific Northwest. The use of Oregon grape root for this purpose eventually spread to the settlers in those areas. Oregon grape root contains the alkaloid berberine, which acts as an antibiotic when used topically.

DIRECTIONS: Place ½ ounce of Oregon grape root in a pot and add one pint of boiling water. Let cool to room temperature. Apply to the eyes with a clean cloth.

EYEBRIGHT

Eyebright (*Euphrasia officinalis*) is a plant native to Europe that traditionally has been used to treat conjunctivitis and other eye infections. It was first listed in British herbals in the 1500s, with the annotation that its flowers look like small yellow eyes. It is used as an eye remedy today in the natural medicine of Appalachia.

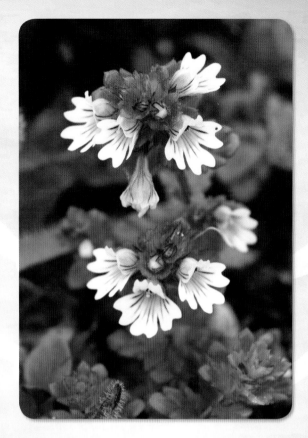

Like many of the other plants in this section, eyebright has both astringent and anti-inflammatory properties that may reduce inflammation in mucous membranes. Eyebright is very drying, so it should be used only on eye conditions that involve mucus or discharge. (It could increase the discomfort of dry, irritated eyes.) For this reason, the use of eyebright for eye problems has been discouraged by some authorities.

Here are directions for using eyebright from a German medical text called *Lehrbuch der Phytotherapie* (*Herbal Medicine*) by R.F. Weiss, M.D. The text is used in German medical and pharmacy schools.

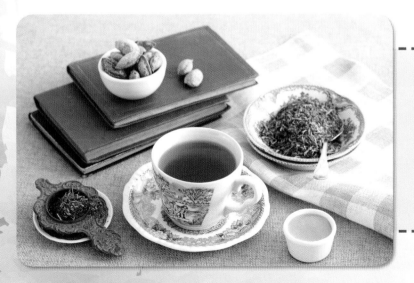

DIRECTIONS: Place one tablespoon of eyebright leaves in one pint of water. Cover and simmer for ten minutes. Strain and apply to the eyes with a clean cloth. At the same time, pour the tea into a cup and drink. Do this twice a day.

GOLDENSEAL

During the second decade of the 19th century, American botanist Constantine Rafinesque traveled among the American Indians of the Ohio River and Mississippi River valleys, recording their uses of plants. His work resulted in *Medical Flora*, the first scientific book of medical botany in the United States. In his research, Rafinesque discovered that the Indians in the Midwest used goldenseal as a specific treatment for sore, inflamed, or infected eyes. They made an eyewash by boiling the root in water. This and other uses for goldenseal were quickly adopted by the European settlers in the eastern United States. A goldenseal eyewash is still used today in the traditions of Appalachia.

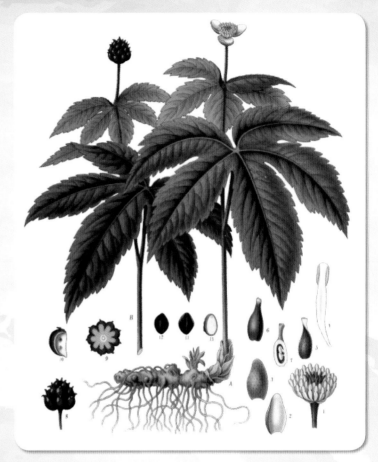

Part of goldenseal's medicinal action on the eyes is due to its constituents hydrastine and berberine. Like several other remedies in this section, it also has an astringent effect on swollen mucous membranes. Goldenseal is an endangered species in this country due to loss of habitat, overharvesting, and widespread use by the American public, who mistakenly take it as a treatment for cold and flu. In fact, treating eye infections is one of the few legitimate medical uses for goldenseal. Because goldenseal is no longer readily available, other berberine-containing herbs, including Oregon grape root, are less expensive, yet still effective, substitutes.

DIRECTIONS: Boil a handful of goldenseal root in one quart of water for twenty minutes. Let cool to room temperature. Apply to the eyes with a clean cloth.

CHRYSANTHEMUM BLOSSOMS

A Chinese treatment for tired, bloodshot, or sore eyes is a tea of dried chrysanthemum flowers.

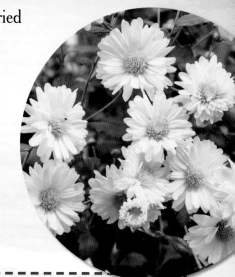

Chrysanthemum (*Chrysanthemum indicum flos.*) is a popular beverage among Asians in the United States and can be found in almost any Asian market. The Chinese name for chrysanthemum is *yeh-chu-hua*, or simply *chu-hua*.

Chinese and Japanese researchers have found constituents in chrysanthemum tea that inhibit *Staphylococcus* bacteria, a common cause of eye infection in some parts of the world. Chrysanthemum is also effective against a wide variety of other bacteria and viruses.

DIRECTIONS: Obtain chrysanthemum flowers from a health food store, herb shop, or Asian market. Purchase the whole dried flowers instead of a prepared tea. (The prepared products usually contain sugar or other additives that are not appropriate to put into the eyes.) Place a large handful of the flowers in a pot and add one quart of boiling water. Cover and steep for ten minutes. Strain, setting aside the still-warm flowers. Drink a cup of the tea. Wrap the still-warm flowers in a clean cloth, and, while lying down, apply to the eyes until the flowers cool.

EYE BATH

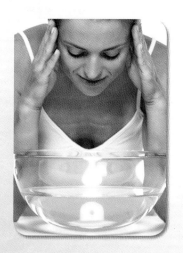

At the turn of the century, German immigrants recommended using an eye bath to remove objects from the eyes.

DIRECTIONS: Use a bowl large enough to completely immerse the face. Fill the bowl with cold water. Open the eyes underwater several times, until the object is washed out. Eye cups are still available in some pharmacies and are very convenient to use.

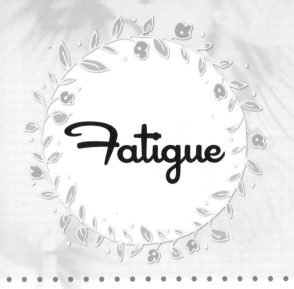

Fatigue

If you suffer from fatigue, try some of the natural remedies below—they're sure to get you moving again in no time.

Fatigue may be physical or mental exhaustion, an overwhelming feeling of weariness, or a lack of energy and enthusiasm for even pleasant activities.

Fatigue is a symptom of a vast number of diseases and disorders. More than 10 million people visit their doctors each year complaining of fatigue, making fatigue the seventh most common reason we make a doctor's appointment for a medical checkup. Between one-fourth and one-fifth of all Americans will seek medical advice for severe or chronic fatigue at some point in their professional lives.

The remedies in this section are appropriate for treating normal, brief periods of fatigue that are the result of some unusual stress or unexpected disruption of sleep. Any severe or long-lasting fatigue requires a medical checkup to determine the cause of stress.

Fatigue and tiring rapidly with minimal activity are often among the early signs of an approaching illness. Fatigue is a warning sign of a variety of diseases and disorders, including the common cold, influenza, hepatitis, infectious mononucleosis, and other infectious diseases; heart disease; lung disorders, such as emphysema; some glandular diseases, such as diabetes; and anemia and nutritional deficiencies. Deficiencies of the minerals magnesium and zinc, the most common mineral deficiencies in the American population (affecting more than half of us), may cause fatigue in some people as well. Deficiencies of chromium, copper, folic acid, manganese, niacin, pantothenic acid, pyridoxine, thiamine, vitamin A, vitamin B12, vitamin C, iron, and potassium may also be responsible. Overwork, either mental or physical, may also cause fatigue, as can psychological disorders or emotional stress. Sugar and caffeine consumption can also result in severe or chronic fatigue in some individuals.

Fatigue is best remedied by treating the physical disorder

or psychological problem that is causing it. Some types of fatigue, particularly those due to physical overexertion, can probably be prevented by getting adequate exercise and rest. The average hours of sleep an American gets each night have been on the decline for the last twenty-five years. We now sleep an average of seven hours a night. That's about an hour less than the average optimal amount of sleep. A third of Americans sleep less than six hours a night; many of them try to catch up by sleeping more on the weekends. A good alternative to sleeping more at night is to squeeze in naps during the day. Several traditions advocate napping on a regular basis to prevent or treat fatigue.

Better Bitter Tonics

In North American herbal traditions, and in the medicine of the 19th century, bitter tonics have been one of the most often prescribed categories of herbs for fatigue and general debility. Bitter tonics are also commonly prescribed for these conditions by conventional physicians in Germany today.

Although these plants possess a mild to strong bitter flavor, they do not have strong medicinal properties. Many act as mild sedatives. The bitter principles in the plants stimulate the secretion of stomach acid and liver bile. Their reputed tonic effects may thus come from improved digestion and nourishment. (Because these herbs stimulate secretions, they are contraindicated if you have heartburn or other kinds of digestive pain.) The most famous of the bitter tonics in North American herbal history are goldthread (*Coptis trifola*), goldenseal (*Hydrastis canadensis*), Oregon grape root (*Mahonia aquifolium, Berberis aquifolium*), yellow dock (*Rumex crispus*), and dandelion root (*Taraxacum officinale*). Goldthread and goldenseal are practically extinct in North America, however. Betony, included in this section, is a common bitter tonic in British herbalism.

Betony

A folk source from 1824, listed in folklorist Clarence Meyer's *American Folk Medicine*, states that betony (*Stachys officinalis*, *Betonica officinalis*) is a good remedy for general debility that arises from disturbed digestion. The original source of this remedy was probably an immigrant from Europe, where betony had been used as a tonic since at least the time of the ancient Romans. In fact, the physician to the Emperor Augustus, who lived at the time of Jesus Christ's birth, listed forty-seven different diseases he thought betony would cure. The herb has remained so valued in Italy that a popular expression there advises you to "Sell your coat and buy betony."

Although betony is widely used in natural medicine in Europe even today, it has never been used to any extent by North American schools of medicine or by professional herbalists in North America. Betony is the first of the herbs in this section to be classified as a bitter tonic. Betony is also reputed to be a sedative, and its most common use in European herbalism today is for treating nervous tension, nervous headache, and accompanying exhaustion. Don't confuse this plant with North American betony (*Pedicularis* spp.), which grows in the mountainous areas of the West. *Pedicularis*, like *Stachys*, is a sedative, but does not have the bitter tonic properties.

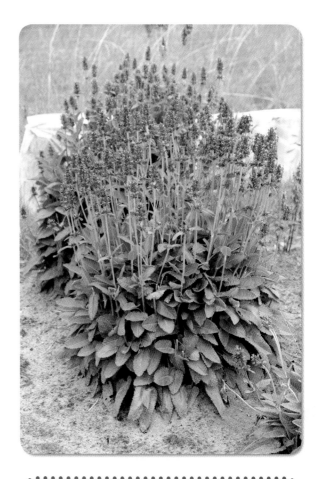

Directions: Place one tablespoon of betony leaves in a one-pint jar and fill with boiling water. Cover and let cool until the water reaches room temperature. Drink the pint in three doses during the day, twenty minutes before meals, for seven to ten days.

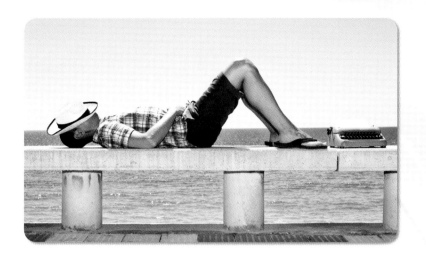

Napping

The Amish have a saying that a half-hour nap in the afternoon is worth two hours of sleep at night. German immigrants at the turn of the century also advocated the afternoon nap, even if for only fifteen minutes, as an important way to restore energy and prevent exhaustion from overwork.

Directions: Take a mid-to-late afternoon nap of fifteen minutes or more, lying down if possible.

Oregon Grape Root

The American Indians of California and the Pacific Northwest used Oregon grape root (*Mahonia aquifolium, Berberis aquifolium*) to treat general debility. The herb acts as a bitter tonic. Although goldthread (*Coptis trifola*) and goldenseal (*Hydrastis canadensis*) are the most famous of the North American bitter tonics, these herbs have become practically extinct on the continent. Oregon grape root has become the most common substitute for these herbs among North American professional herbalists. Its action on the digestive system is due to its bitter alkaloid berberine, which is also present in gold-thread and goldenseal.

Directions: Place one tablespoon of Oregon grape root in one pint of water. Cover the pot and simmer for twenty minutes. Let cool to room temperature. Drink one ounce of the tea twenty minutes before meals for one to three weeks.

Fatigue

Asian Ginseng

Asian ginseng (*Panax ginseng*) has probably been used in Chinese natural medicine since about 3000 BC and remains the most famous and sought after herbal remedy in Chinese culture. In contemporary Chinese medicine, ginseng is used to restore strength when there is physical weakness or exhaustion resulting from a long-term illness. It is also used in natural medicine throughout the modern cities of China, Korea, Japan, and Southeast Asia to increase the individual's ability to resist the stresses of modern life.

Asian ginseng has been used in the natural medicine of Asian communities in North America for at least the last century. In the United States, it entered into mainstream society first through the counterculture movement of the 1960s and 1970s and then through the health food trade and the current natural healing movement.

Don't take Asian ginseng unless you are run down, because it can be over stimulating for a person with a normal energy level. Don't take it for chronic fatigue without first getting a thorough medical checkup, because the energy boost from the ginseng may simply temporarily mask the symptoms of a nutritional deficiency or a more serious underlying disease. And don't take ginseng if you also habitually use caffeine. If you begin to experience neck tension, insomnia, increased menstrual flow, or headaches, stop taking ginseng. Prolonged use after experiencing such symptoms can cause high blood pressure.

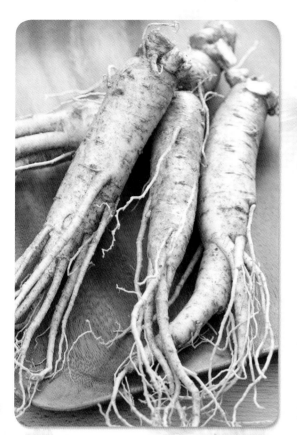

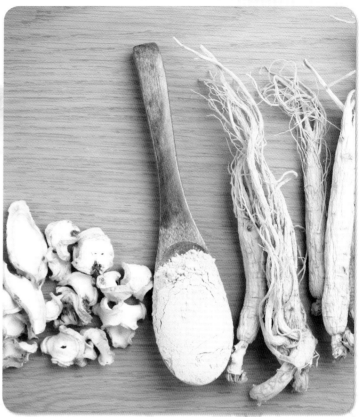

Directions: Purchase a commercial ginseng product in a reputable herb shop. You'll generally find better quality ginseng there than in a health food store, supermarket, or pharmacy. Don't skimp on price—the more expensive products are usually the better quality products. Take one to two grams of ginseng powder a day, in two or three doses, for six weeks at a time. Take a two week break every six weeks.

Also, you can buy some whole ginseng roots—roots of average quality cost about $180 a pound in herb shops. An individual root costs between $6 and $12. Chop four ounces of the ginseng root and place in a quart of liquor such as vodka. Cover and let stand for five or six weeks in a cool dark place, turning the jar frequently. Don't strain. Take one ounce of the liquid each day, midmorning or just before lunch.

Fatigue

Siberian Ginseng

Siberian ginseng (*Eleutherococcus senticosus, Acanthopanax senticosus*) has been used in Chinese medicine since the birth of Jesus Christ, but its properties as an adaptogen were not clearly identified until after World War II. Russian ginseng researchers investigated the Siberian ginseng plant, looking for a less expensive alternative to Asian ginseng. Both animal and human trials showed that the plant increased response and adaptation to stress. The Siberian ginseng preparation remains a popular medicine in Russia today and is available over-the-counter. It is also sometimes prescribed by doctors in Europe.

The term Siberian ginseng was invented by marketers trying to sell the product in the United States in the 1970s, hoping to capitalize on the popularity of Asian ginseng. Siberian ginseng thus entered the folklore of North America through health food stores, and is now widely used in every region of the country. It is important to note that the *Eleutherococcus* plant is not actually a "ginseng," however, and it is nowhere near as powerful as Asian ginseng. But it is also less likely to cause overstimulation, insomnia, high blood pressure, or other side effects common to Asian ginseng. Because of its mildness, it is better suited for the average American than is Asian ginseng.

Unfortunately, much of the Siberian ginseng on the market is adulterated. The Canadian government recently examined three shipments arriving from Asia and found that two of them contained no *Eleutherococcus* at all; the other did, but also had five percent caffeine added. Most American products are also not made according to the specifications of the Russians and are weak by comparison to the Russian products, sometimes with only one-fifth the strength. For the best products, made according to the specifications of the Russian pharmacopoeia, look for a description such as "1:1 extract in 30% alcohol" on the label of the tincture bottle.

Directions: Find a product matching the "1:1" description, and take a dropperful of the tincture three times a day for up to six weeks. Take a two-week break before starting another course of treatment.

150

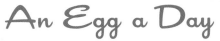

An Egg a Day

Folklorist Clarence Meyer's collection of traditional American remedies called *American Folk Medicine* advises taking an egg a day to restore strength in cases of debility. Deficiencies of several nutrients—including iron, vitamin A, folic acid, riboflavin, and pantothenic acid—may cause fatigue. A single egg contains significant amounts of these nutrients.

Directions: Beat a raw egg, flavor with a little sugar or honey, and drink it. If the texture is not appetizing, blend the egg in a glass of milk and drink it that way.

Note: Some people caution that a raw egg may be contaminated with *salmonella* and should be cooked before eating.

Adaptogens

An entire class of Chinese herbs—ginseng being the most famous of them—are used to restore the weary. These herbs and their beneficial actions were made more accessible to Westerners when Russian researchers investigated them in the decades after World War II. In fact, it was the Russians who coined the term *adaptogen*. An adaptogen helps you "adapt" to different kinds of stress, whether from cold weather, overwork, or staying

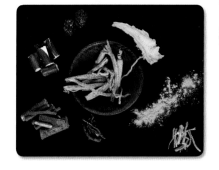

up at night with a crying baby. The Russians verified this adaptogen property in Asian ginseng, Siberian ginseng, schizandra berries, and several other herbs. Although they have been used in Asian communities in North America for more than a hundred years, these plants are now popular in various other communities throughout the United States as well. In fact, you can purchase various kinds of ginseng today in most pharmacies and supermarkets.

Fatigue

FEVER

To understand what having a fever means, its helps to know something about how your body controls temperature. There is quite a range in what is considered "normal" in body temperature. (As you know, everyone has a temperature; when it rises above what is considered normal and stays there, it is then termed a fever.)

The average human body temperature falls between 98 degrees Fahrenheit and 98.6 degrees Fahrenheit during daily activities, but normal temperatures can range anywhere between 97 and 99 degrees Fahrenheit. (And many healthy active children have normal temperatures as high as 99 to 101 degrees Fahrenheit.) Your normal body temperature fluctuates about half a degree during the day, with the lowest reading usually occurring in the early morning and the highest in the late afternoon. The body temperature can be elevated to a range of 101 to 105 degrees Fahrenheit during fever (or during heavy exercise) and may also fall by about a degree below normal with exposure to cold.

152

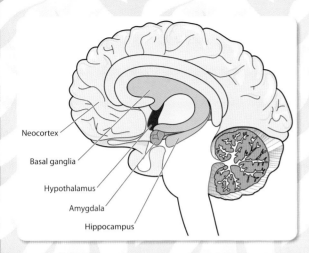

Neocortex

Basal ganglia

Hypothalamus

Amygdala

Hippocampus

Fever is regulated by a control center in the brain called the hypothalamus. The fever is activated when the hypothalamus senses tiny amounts of bacteria or bacterial toxins in the blood. The hypothalamus may also recognize chemical triggers in the blood that are sent out by white blood cells engaged in fighting off the infection.

The hypothalamus is like the thermostat in your house—it is set for a certain temperature range. When it recognizes an infection or immune response, it turns the temperature up. Blood is shunted from the exterior of the body to the interior. As a result, the muscles may involuntarily shiver in order to replace the lost heat. Like a factory suddenly turned up to maximum production, the body's metabolism speeds up by as much as thirty percent in order to produce more white blood cells, antibodies, and other elements of the immune system. Once the infection is successfully fought off, the hypothalamus turns the thermostat back down and the body sweats to cool off.

Early in the 20th century, conventional doctors routinely suppressed all fevers with aspirin or related drugs. Modern medicine now recognizes that a fever is a beneficial healing response and mild fevers are no longer routinely suppressed. (Any fever that reaches 104 degrees Fahrenheit or lasts more than three days requires prompt medical attention, however.) The best natural treatment for a simple fever is to support the body's response. Resting in bed, keeping warm, drinking plenty of liquids, and avoiding solid food helps the body to do its job to fight off the infection. Many of the natural remedies below help to induce a sweat to cool a fever.

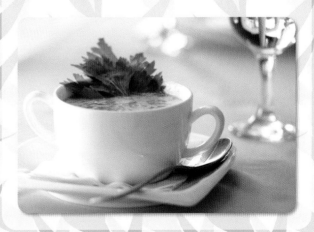

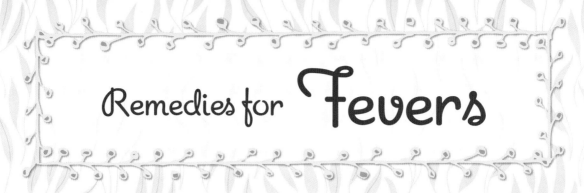

Remedies for Fevers

Ginger

A fever remedy popular in New England, Appalachia, North Carolina, Indiana, and China is ginger tea. Ginger tea is used to lower fever in the traditional medical systems of India and Arabia as well. Ginger (*Zingiber officinale*) induces sweating, which helps to cool the body during fever. It also contains many anti-inflammatory compounds, including some with mild aspirin-like effects. Thus, ginger may lower fever in more ways than one—it has both diaphoretic and anti-inflammatory effects. Several of these constituents in ginger have also shown to lower fever in animals.

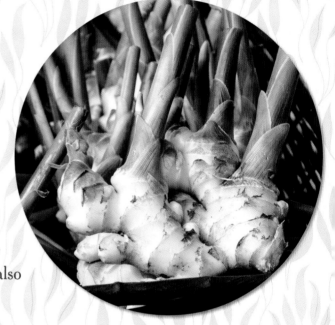

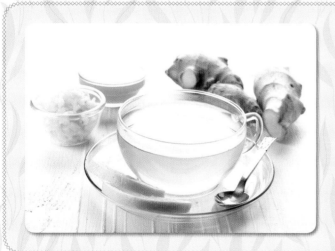

Directions: Thinly slice a fresh ginger root (the root should be about the size of your thumb). Place the ginger in one quart of water. Bring to a boil, then simmer on the lowest possible heat for thirty minutes in a covered pot. Let cool for thirty more minutes. Strain and drink up to one cup, sweetened with honey. Repeat three times a day as desired. As a precaution, don't take ginger in this dosage during pregnancy.

Peppermint

Peppermint (*Mentha piperita*) is a natural remedy used for fever in Indiana and by some Hispanics in the Southwest. In China, cornmint (*Mentha arvensis*), a close relative of peppermint, is used in the same manner. Both plants, when taken as a hot tea, induce sweating, and help to cool a fever. Cornmint and peppermint also contain large amounts of antiseptic and cooling menthol. In addition, as the steamy hot tea is drunk and the fragrance is inhaled, the menthol may act as a decongestant. Thus, this treatment might be best for treating fever accompanied by congestion.

Directions: Place ½ ounce of peppermint leaves in a one-quart jar. Fill with boiling water and cover tightly. Let steep twenty minutes. While fever persists, strain and drink two or three cups a day. Wrap yourself in blankets and rest in bed after each cup.

Catnip

A fever remedy from the Seventh Day Adventists calls for drinking catnip tea while soaking the feet in hot water. Catnip (*Nepeta cataria*) is also a fever remedy in the folk traditions of New England and Appalachia. Catnip's warming aromatic substances are diaphoretic and help to induce a sweat. (Sticking the feet in hot water can induce sweating as well.) Catnip also purportedly acts as a sedative and may help you to rest and relax.

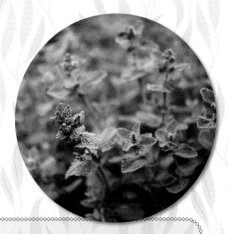

Directions: Fill the bathtub or a smaller tub with hot water. Put the feet in the water while drinking the hot tea. (This remedy is contraindicated in diabetics because of the possibility of burning the feet.)

To make the tea, pour boiling water over one ounce of catnip leaves in a one-quart jar. Cover tightly and let steep for ten to fifteen minutes. As the fever persists, soak your feet every three to four hours while drinking half a cup of the tea.

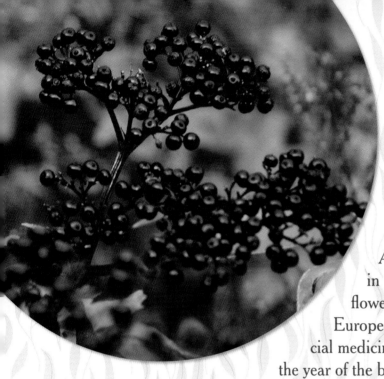

Elder Flowers & Berries

Black elder (*Sambucus nigra*) is a famous flu and fever remedy from European traditional medicine. The plant's medicinal uses date back to the ancient Romans. Related elder species are native to North America. The Paiute and Shoshone Indians in the Rocky Mountains used the leaves and flowers of their local species for fevers, just as the Europeans used black elder. Elderberry was an official medicine in the United States Pharmacopoeia from the year of the book's founding in 1820 until 1909. The use of elder flower tea for fevers is still recorded in the natural medicine of the Amish, as well as in Indiana and by Hispanics in the Southwest.

The standard German medical textbook *Lehrbuch der Phytotherapie* describes elder as an immune stimulant. Elder flower tea is approved by the German government as a medicine for colds accompanied by cough. Recent research in Israel and Panama show that elderberry juice stimulates the immune system and can also significantly reduce the duration of an influenza attack.

The flowers contain anti-inflammatory constituents. (These constituents may also be present in other parts of the plant but have not yet been measured there. The bark and root of elder are very strong laxatives and should be avoided.) The flowers are traditionally taken as a tea, while the berries are made into syrups. Taking too much elder tea, however, whether in the form of flowers or berries, can bring about a feeling of nausea.

Directions: Place ½ ounce of elder flowers in a one-quart canning jar. Fill with boiling water. Cover and let steep for twenty minutes. Strain and pour a cup. Sweeten with honey. Take a cup every four hours for a fever, especially one accompanying the flu. Wrap yourself in warm blankets after drinking the tea. If the tea gives you a queasy feeling after a few doses, take less or stop taking it all together to ease the feeling.

Lemon Balm

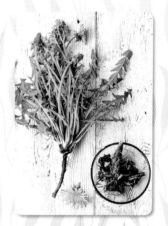

In Indiana, lemon balm (*Melissa officinalis*) is a remedy for fever. The plant, which was native to southern Europe and northern Africa, arrived with the colonists and spread throughout North America. It has been used as a relaxing and sweat-inducing herb at least since the 12th century in Germany, where it is approved today as a medicine for digestive complaints or sleeping disorders, though not specifically for fevers. Of the sweat-inducing herbs included in this section, lemon balm is probably the mildest herb and is the most suitable for use in children. Lemon balm is also a mild sedative and can help relax the restless patient with cold or flu.

Directions: Pour boiling water over one teaspoon of the dried herb in a cup. Fill and let steep for ten minutes. While the tea is steeping, inhale the steam from the cup. Strain and drink the tea, sweetened with honey as desired, up to four cups a day.

Dandelion

A common herb used to reduce fever in Chinese medicine is dandelion. (In traditional Chinese medicine, dandelion is classified as a "heat clearing" herb.) The Chinese dandelion (*Taraxacum mongolici*) and this country's common backyard dandelion (*Taraxacum officinale*) have similar appearances and constituents. Like many of the herbs in this category, dandelion contains several anti-inflammatory constituents. But, unlike the other herbs listed above, dandelion does not induce sweating. Its fever-reducing activity, if any, comes from some other mechanism. Dandelion has not been tested for fever-lowering properties by conventional scientists.

Directions: Pick some dandelions, taking the whole root and leaf. (Be sure to harvest them away from lawns or fields that may have been sprayed with chemical pesticides.) Wash the roots well with running water. Place two ounces of the plant in one quart of water. Bring to a boil and cover. Simmer on the lowest heat for thirty to forty minutes. When suffering from fever, drink the quart in four doses during the course of a day. If your fever is not better within three days, be sure to see a doctor. Don't take dandelion if you suffer from indigestion or heartburn.

Fever

Willow Bark

The Greeks used willow bark (*Salix* spp.) to treat pain more than 2,400 years ago. American Indians of the Alabama, Chickasaw, Houma, Montagnais, Shoshone, and Thompson tribes and the Ninivak Eskimos were using willow bark for the same purpose before the arrival of the European colonists. Scientific investigations of willow bark during the 19th century led to the isolation of its pain-relieving and fever-lowering constituents, and, ultimately, to the synthesis of aspirin in 1898. (Willow bark itself does not contain aspirin, but similar milder compounds.)

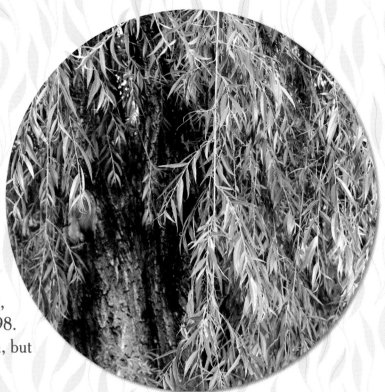

Willow bark is used to lower fever or reduce pain in the natural medicine of Indiana, New England, and the Southwest, as well as by professional medical herbalists of North America and Britain. The German government has approved the use of willow bark by its conventional physicians for treating pain and fever. Besides its aspirin-like constituent salicin, willow bark contains other anti-inflammatory constituents as well.

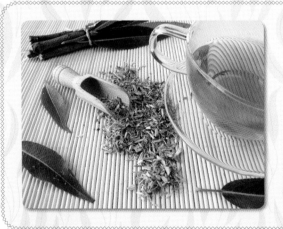

Directions: Purchase some willow bark capsules in a health food store or herb shop. Take as directed on the label. Alternately, place two teaspoons of powdered willow bark in a cup, fill with boiling water, and let steep for fifteen to twenty minutes. Sweeten with honey as desired, and drink up to four cups a day for as long as the fever persists.

Willow Bark

American Ginseng

Another herb used to treat feverish illnesses in Chinese medicine is American ginseng (*Panax quinquefolium*). It is also used by residents of Appalachia.

Although American ginseng has never been used much in American medicine, it is a very popular remedy in China. Hundreds of tons of American ginseng are shipped from farms in Michigan and Wisconsin to China every year. (American ginseng, also reputed for its sedating effects, is often more popular than Asian ginseng in Chinatowns throughout North America.) The Chinese use the American ginseng species for different purposes than their own native Asian ginseng (*Panax ginseng*). They view American ginseng as a "cooling" plant; they take it during hot summer weather and to cool feverish illnesses. Other than the basic identification of its constituents, very little scientific research has investigated American ginseng. Its "cooling" properties have not been examined or demonstrated.

Directions: Chop three ounces of ginseng and place in one quart of liquor. Cover and let stand for five or six weeks in a cool dark place, turning the jar frequently. When fighting a fever, take one ounce after dinner or before bed.

Lemon

Lemons in the form of hot lemonade is a natural remedy for fever and influenza in New England and Indiana. The ancient Romans used lemons in the same way. No one has performed clinical trials to see if this method really works, but the constituents of lemon and its fragrant oils may indeed be helpful for treating fever and infection.

Lemon juice is an expectorant, increasing the flow of healthy mucus to infected mucous membranes. Other constituents of lemon are antimicrobial and anti-inflammatory. It is not known whether clinically significant levels of these constituents are present in hot lemonade, however.

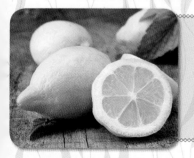

Directions: Pour one cup of boiling water over a blended whole lemon—skin, pulp, and all. Let the mixture steep for five minutes. While the tea is steeping, inhale the fumes. Drink one cup. Do this at first onset of a fever, and repeat three to four times a day for the duration of the infection.

Fever

HEADACHES

If you are prone to headache pain, read on.
The remedies that follow can help you feel better—fast.

A headache is a symptom of disease, and not a disease in itself. Rarely is a headache the symptom of a serious illness—most headaches are caused by minor conditions, such as muscle tension in the neck and around the skull or inflammation of blood vessels in the brain.

There are three basic types of headaches. The vascular headache occurs when blood vessels in the head enlarge and press on nerves, causing pain. The most common vascular headache is the migraine. The second type of headache is the muscle contraction headache, which results when the muscles of the face, neck, or scalp contract and tighten. A tension headache is an example of a muscle contraction headache. The third kind of headache is the inflammatory headache. Such a headache is the result of pressure within the head. The causes range from relatively minor conditions, such as sinusitis, to more serious problems, such as brain tumors.

Headaches are most often treated with aspirin and nonsteroidal anti-inflammatory drugs (NSAIDs) such as ibuprofen or acetaminophen. Treatment of a migraine already in progress usually consists of a

Using Your Head

A German herbal that was used by turn-of-the-century immigrants suggested binding mint across the forehead, a practice that American Indians also used for treating headache pain. Traditions from every region of North America and Europe recommend applying substances to the head to treat headaches. For example, from New England to the Southwest, remedies suggest applying camphor spirits and vinegar to the head to treat headache pain. In New England, practitioners of natural medicine apply witch hazel to the forehead or spread sauerkraut on the temples. Other North American traditions call for applying raw onions or boneset leaves to the forehead. We don't know if any these methods really work, but some medicinal substances, such as the anti-inflammatory rosmarinic acid found in mint, are easily absorbed through the skin.

drug therapy program chosen from a variety of painkillers, sedatives, and special drugs and remedies, including vasoconstricting drugs and caffeine. Tension headaches can be treated by eliminating the tension or correcting the physical problem that is causing the headaches. This can sometimes be done through physical manipulation of the spine or skull by a chiropractic or osteopathic physician.

The herbal remedies for headaches, which are still used today by alternative physicians in the United States and by some conventional doctors in Europe, fall into four categories: pain-relievers, anti-inflammatories, sedatives, and digestive herbs. The pain-relieving and anti-inflammatory herbs may relieve most types of headaches. The sedatives work well for relieving tension headaches. The digestive herbs and laxatives are most useful for treating headaches that accompany digestive sluggishness or constipation.

Where Aspirin Came From

Aspirin is perhaps the best-known drug for treating headaches in North America today. In fact, per-capita consumption of aspirin in the United States is one tablet per person per week. Aspirin was "discovered" after chemists studied plants such as willow bark, sage, and pennyroyal. These plants, and others, have traditionally been used to treat pain.

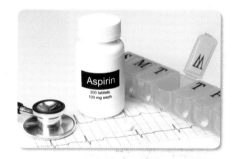

The first of the plants to be studied was willow bark, which had been used by both the ancient Greeks and by the American Indians to treat pain. The pain-relieving constituent of willow bark, salicin, was isolated in the 19th century. Similar aspirin-like compounds were later found in other plants as well. In fact, chemists created acetylsalicylic acid—aspirin—from salicylic acid obtained from meadowsweet.

Further study in the 20th century has led to a whole new class of drugs, called nonsteroidal anti-inflammatory drugs (NSAIDs), which have anti-inflammatory properties similar to those of aspirin. NSAIDs are useful in the treatment of athletic injuries, postoperative pain, rheumatoid and osteoarthritis, and skin, bone, and teeth disorders. We owe our knowledge of this new class of medicines to the original medicinal use of plants for pain.

Headaches

Remedies for *Headaches*

Willow Bark

More than 2,400 years ago, the Greeks used willow bark (*Salix* spp.) to treat headache pain. American Indians of the Alabama, Chickasaw, Houma, Montagnais, Shoshone, and Thompson tribes and the Ninivak Eskimos used it for the same purpose, even before the arrival of the European colonists. Willow bark is still used to treat headache pain in the medicine of Indiana, New England, and the Southwest. It is recommended by professional medical herbalists of North America and Great Britain. The German government has approved its use by conventional physicians for treating pain and fever.

The most important active constituent in willow bark is salicin, but the bark also contains at least three other anti-inflammatory constituents. In Germany, the suggested dose is about one gram of the powdered bark—the amount in about two average-sized gelatin capsules. Willow bark is not as potent as aspirin, but it is less likely to cause stomach upset.

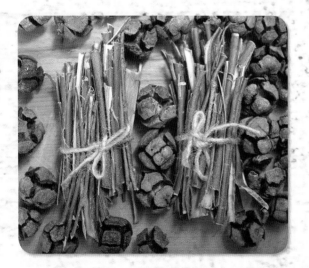

Directions: To make a tea, place two teaspoons of powdered willow bark in a cup and fill with boiling water. Let steep for fifteen to twenty minutes. Sweeten with honey as desired. Drink up to four cups a day. Note that salicin can cause skin rashes in some people.

Alternately, you can purchase willow bark capsules in a health food store or an herb shop. Take as directed on the product label.

Rosemary-Sage Tea

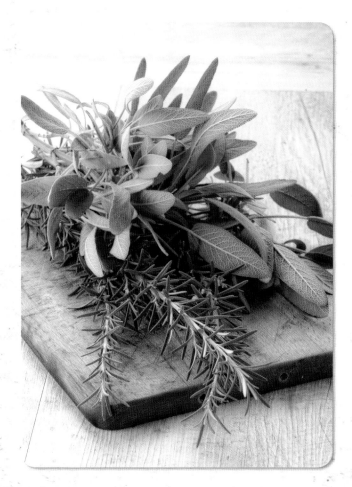

A natural remedy for treating headache pain is to drink a tea of rosemary (*Rosmarinus officinalis*) and sage (*Salvia officinalis*). Rosemary has been a popular medicine in Europe for treating pain at least since the time of the ancient Greeks. Among the Greeks, rosemary had a reputation for improving the memory.

Today, rosemary is used to soothe headaches in the traditional medicine of China, and, in the United States, it is used for the same purpose in Indiana and among the Amish. The German government has approved the use of rosemary for pain. There, rosemary is often used externally, in preparations such as salves and baths. It is a common folk use to apply rosemary to the temples in the form of a poultice to relieve headache pain.

Sage is not often used in natural medicine as a pain reliever, but it has an important chemical constituent in common with rosemary—rosmarinic acid. In addition, the combination of rosemary and sage contains more than twenty anti-inflammatory constituents, although some of these exist only in minute amounts. Seek medical attention for any headache that lasts longer than three days. Do not ingest rosemary in any amount exceeding those usually found in foods because of the herb's reputed abortifacient and emmenagogue effects.

Directions: Place one teaspoon of crushed rosemary leaves and one teaspoon of crushed sage leaves in a cup. Fill with boiling water. Cover well to prevent the escape of volatile substances. Let steep until the tea reaches room temperature. Take ½-cup doses two or three times a day for two or three days. You don't have to mix rosemary and sage to find pain relief. You can also try drinking either rosemary or sage teas separately.

Headaches

American Pennyroyal

Pennyroyal tea (*Hedeoma pulegioides*) is a headache remedy of the Onondaga Indians. In European medicine, a European species of pennyroyal (*Mentha pulegioides L.*) is used for pain relief. In fact, the 17th century British herbalist John Gerard wrote of pennyroyal: "A Garland of Pennie Royall made and worne about the head is of great force against swimming in the head, and the paines and giddiness thereof." The use of pennyroyal for treating headaches persists today in the natural medicine of Appalachia and Indiana. Pennyroyal contains significant amounts of the anti-inflammatory substance diosmin.

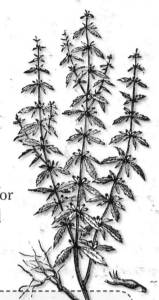

Directions: Place one teaspoon of dried pennyroyal leaves in a cup and fill with boiling water. Cover well to avoid the loss of volatile constituents. Let steep. Take ½-cup doses as desired, up to four times a day. Seek medical attention for any headache that lasts longer than three days.

Yarrow

Yarrow (*Achillea millefolium*) has been used as a universal pain and headache remedy among various American Indian tribes, including the Cheyenne, Chippewa, Gosuite, Iroquois, Lummi, Mendocino, Navaho, Paiute, Seneca, and Shoshone. Yarrow contains at least eighteen anti-inflammatory constituents, including salicylic acid, an aspirin-like substance.

Directions: Place one ounce of dried or fresh yarrow leaves in a one-quart jar and fill with boiling water. Cover tightly to prevent the escape of the aromatic constituents. The dose is one-half cup of the tea, two to four times a day. If any headache persists for more than three days, see your doctor.

Coffee or Tea

Coffee or tea is recommended as a headache cure in several traditions. Caffeine is the medicinal constituent responsible for the benefits. Caffeine is also used in conventional medicine to treat migraine headaches. It works by constricting the vessels of the brain, which are sometimes dilated during a headache attack. Tea is recommended in New England, and strong black coffee in Appalachia. Black coffee is a famous cure throughout Europe and North America for the type of headache that accompanies hangover. Note that habitual use of caffeine can cause headache on withdrawal, however.

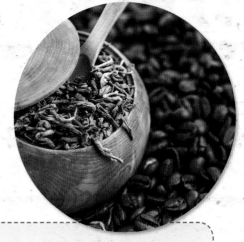

Directions: Make a pot of strong black coffee or tea and drink two cups to relieve an acute headache.

Laxatives

A collection of remedies by folklorist Clarence Meyer called *American Folk Medicine* suggests taking low doses of laxatives to cure a headache. This remedy is best used on headaches that accompany constipation. The habitual use of laxatives is not recommended, however.

Directions: Place ¼ teaspoon of senna leaves in a cup. Add ¼ teaspoon of sage leaves and ¼ teaspoon of powdered ginger. Fill the cup with boiling water. Let steep until cool. Drink a cup every four hours. Do not exceed three doses in a day. Do not repeat the treatment for a second day. If the constipation and headache persist, see a physician. Do not use laxatives during pregnancy.

Mints

The mints—peppermint (*Mentha piperita*) and spearmint (*mentha spicata*)—are used as headache remedies in the medicine of the particular regions where they grow. American Indians of both eastern and western North America, including the Cherokee, Iroquois, Gosuite, and Paiute tribes, used these mints as headache remedies. Some tribes crushed the plant and inhaled the fumes; others placed the plant on the forehead or temples in the same way rosemary is used.

Peppermint

Spearmint

Today, mints are used in the medicine of China, Mexico, Appalachia, and the American Southwest to treat headaches. The mints contain about the same levels of the anti-inflammatory rosmarinic acid as do rosemary and sage.

Directions: Place one ounce of dried mint leaves in a one-quart jar and fill with boiling water. Cover tightly to prevent the escape of the aromatic constituents. The dose is ½ cup of tea, two to four times a day. If a headache persists for more than three days, a visit to the doctor is in order.

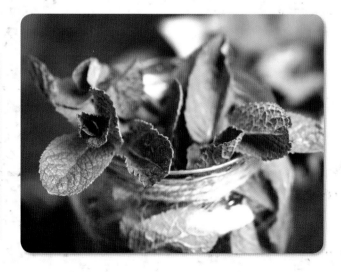

166

Wormwood

Plants of the *Artemisia* genus (*Artemisia* spp.) have been used as pain remedies by at least twenty-two American Indian tribes throughout North America. Some tribes received the pain-relieving properties of the plants by burning them and inhaling their smoke and aromatic oils. To treat a headache, others made a tea of the leaves and used them as a wash on the forehead and temples. The use of the *Artemisia* species is recorded today in the natural medicine of northern New Mexico. The European species *Artemisia absinthum* (or wormwood) is approved as a digestive stimulant by the German government. Excessive use in large amounts can lead to brain damage, however.

The active constituents of plants in the *Artemisia* species include bitter digestive stimulants and anti-inflammatory volatile oils such as azulenes. These constituents are also present in yarrow and chamomile.

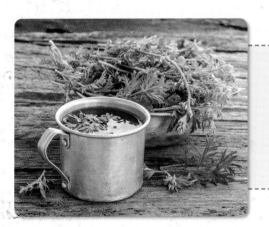

Directions: Place one teaspoon of wormwood leaves in a cup of water and fill with boiling water. Cover well. Let cool to room temperature. Take ½-cup doses every three hours for up to three days. If the headache persists, see a doctor.

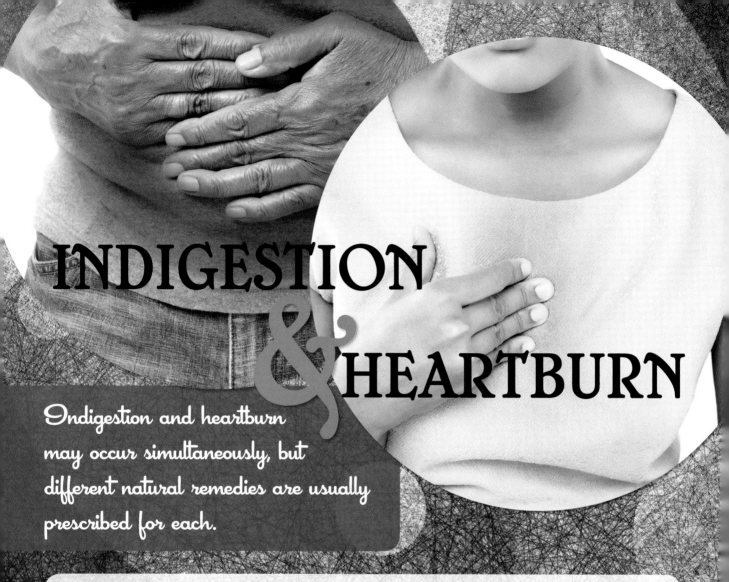

INDIGESTION & HEARTBURN

Indigestion and heartburn may occur simultaneously, but different natural remedies are usually prescribed for each.

Painful indigestion and heartburn are so common in the United States today that antacids are among the top-selling categories of over-the-counter drugs. This section deals with digestive pain rather than sluggish, inefficient digestion. Although the two conditions may occur simultaneously, different remedies are usually prescribed for each. For instance, bitter herbs are commonly prescribed for sluggish digestion, but they are contraindicated if pain is present. Bitter herbs increase the secretion of digestive juices, which increases pain.

Simple digestive pain can come from two main causes: inflammation of the wall of the stomach or intestine, or spasms of the intestinal muscles, often in response to a buildup of gas. The most common causes of digestive inflammation are irritation of the digestive lining by the body's own digestive secretions, infection by a bacterium known as *Helicobacter pylori*, or irritation by offending foods. Persistent indigestion pain should be a cue to visit the doctor, who will help you experiment with your diet to determine and remove the cause.

Heartburn—a gassy, burning sensation in your upper abdomen, sometimes accompanied by the regurgitation of sour, bitter material into your throat or mouth—actually has nothing to do with your heart. Heartburn indicates that the lower part of your esophagus, the upper part of your stomach, or the first section of your bowel has become irritated, and the contents of your stomach have started to back up into the esophagus. Most cases of heartburn aren't serious. The easiest way to avoid a simple case of heartburn? Moderation. Heartburn is generally the result of eating too much too fast.

Eating while under stress is also a major cause of indigestion and heartburn. When relaxed, the body secretes its own antacids from the pancreas and bile ducts in response to food entering the intestine. In a state of stress, these secretions shut off. Thus "acid" indigestion may not be due to excess acid, but to a deficiency of the neutralizing secretions. The best way to turn these secretions back on is to relax for at least ten minutes before eating. Persistent inflammation of the digestive tract can cause ulceration. Ulcers can have serious and even fatal complications if they bleed or if the ulcer eats entirely through the intestine.

The most common categories of natural remedies for digestive pain and heartburn are demulcent herbs (slimy mucilaginous plants that coat and soothe inflamed tissue), herbs containing anti-inflammatory substances, and carminative herbs, which reduce the spasms of intestinal cramps that often accompany gas.

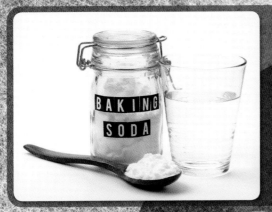

Baking Soda

A do-it-yourself antacid remedy of questionable safety from various streams of North American is to ingest baking soda. Habitual consumption of large amounts of baking soda can cause salt imbalances in the body, however. A safer method is to use commercial antacids, which contain measured amounts of bicarbonate and provide instructions for safe use on the label.

Slippery Elm

Slippery elm bark (*Ulmus fulva*) is used in modern European and North American professional medical herbalism as a soothing treatment for gastritis and ulcers of the digestive tract. The bark, when mixed with water, makes a slimy mucilaginous mass that is soothing to inflamed tissues. Please note that ulcers can cause internal bleeding and have serious health consequences. If you suffer from ulcers, be sure to see a doctor.

Directions: Place one tablespoon of powdered slippery elm bark in a cup. Fill with boiling water. Let steep for ten minutes. Stir, without straining, and drink the whole cup. Do this as needed for pain.

Caraway Seeds

North Americans know caraway seeds (*Carum carvi*) as the tiny seeds coating the crust of rye bread. Caraway seeds are known throughout the Arabic world and in European natural medicine as a treatment for painful intestinal gas. The German government has approved caraway as an official medicine for that condition. The seeds are used for the same purpose in the medicine of North Carolina, Appalachia, and Indiana.

Directions: Place one teaspoon of crushed caraway seeds in a cup and add boiling water. Cover the cup and let stand for ten minutes. Strain and drink three cups of warm tea a day on an empty stomach. Alternately, you can simply chew on the seeds. Repeat as desired.

Ginger

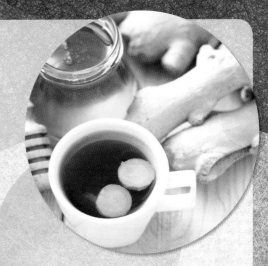

Ginger (*Zingiber officinalis*) is a near-universal remedy for pain in the digestive tract, appearing in the folklore of New England, North Carolina, the southern Appalachians, Indiana, the Southwest, and China. The plant contains both antispasmodic and anti-inflammatory constituents. It also contains topical anesthetic compounds that may directly reduce pain in the digestive tract. In clinical trials ginger has shown to be effective in treating some kinds of nausea.

Directions: Thinly slice a fresh ginger root. (The root should be about the size of your thumb.) Place the slices in one quart of water. Bring to a boil, and then simmer on the lowest possible heat for thirty minutes in a covered pot. Let cool for thirty minutes more. Strain and drink one cup, sweetened with honey as desired.

If you don't have fresh ginger, stir ½ teaspoon of ground ginger into one cup of hot water. Let stand for two to three minutes. Strain and drink, as desired.

Fennel

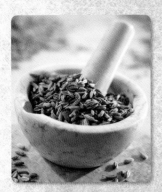

Today, in the professional medical herbalism of Great Britain, North America, and New Zealand, fennel (*Foeniculum vulgare*) is a commonly prescribed herb for abdominal cramping and gas in adults. It appears in the folk medicine of both New England and China. Fennel is an approved medicine in Germany for mild gastrointestinal complaints. It contains sixteen chemical constituents with antispasmodic properties.

Directions: Crush or grind one teaspoon of fennel seeds with a mortar and pestle or coffee grinder. Place the seeds in a cup and fill with boiling water. Cover and let sit ten minutes. Strain and drink three cups of the warm tea each day on an empty stomach.

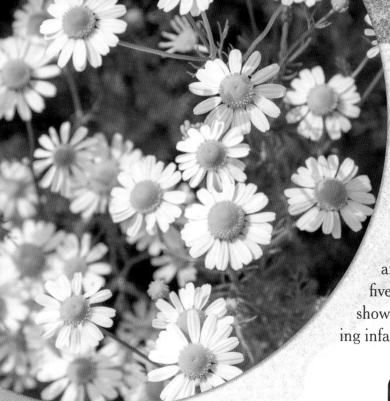

Chamomile

Chamomile (*Matricaria recutita, Anthemis nobilis*) is a popular remedy for treating stomachaches in New England, Indiana, and the Southwest. It is an approved medicine for this purpose in Germany. Chamomile contains at least nineteen antispasmodic constituents as well as five sedative ones. A 1993 clinical trial showed that the plant was effective in relieving infant colic as well.

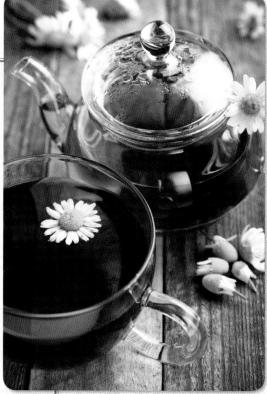

Directions: Place one tablespoon of chamomile flowers in a cup and add boiling water. Cover the cup and let stand for ten minutes. Strain and drink warm three times a day on an empty stomach. Do this for two to three weeks, and then take a break for a week or two. Note: In general, chamomile poses no health threat. If you have suffered previous anaphylactic shock reactions from ragweed, however, talk to your doctor before using this herb.

Mints

Different types of mints, including peppermint and spearmint, are recommended for indigestion in the literature of New England, New York, North Carolina, Appalachia, Indiana, New Mexico, and California. Mints have also been used as carminatives by members of at least seven major North American Indian tribes. Mint is an official digestive aid in German medicine. Peppermint contains antispasmodic compounds. (It is better suited to treating abdominal cramping than heartburn. It can sometimes make heartburn worse.)

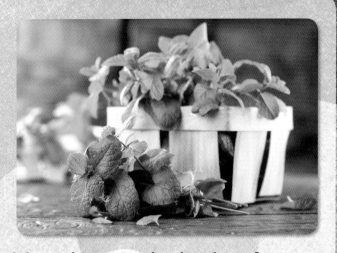

Directions: Place one teaspoon of the dried herb in a cup and add boiling water. Cover the cup and let steep for ten minutes. Strain well and drink one cup three times a day on an empty stomach. Do this as often as desired.

Formula

The following formula, from contemporary North American professional medical herbalism, combines four of the remedies in this section.

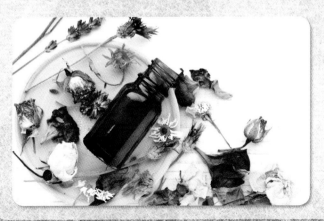

Directions: Place one tablespoon each of chamomile flowers, mint leaves, fennel seeds, and slippery elm bark in a one-pint jar. Fill the jar with boiling water and cover. Let stand until the water reaches room temperature, shaking the bottle occasionally to mix its contents. Strain and drink the quart during the course of the day (on an empty stomach) between meals. Do this as often as desired.

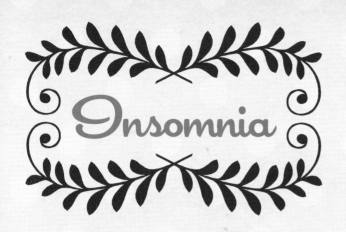

Insomnia

If disturbed sleep leaves you feeling fatigued and not up to par the next day, you may be suffering from insomnia. Here's how to get some shut-eye.

At some point in our lives, between one third and one half of all Americans have a serious bout of chronic insomnia, which is the inability to sleep the desired amount at least three nights a week for a month or more. Insomnia may mean difficulty falling asleep, waking up periodically during the night, or waking

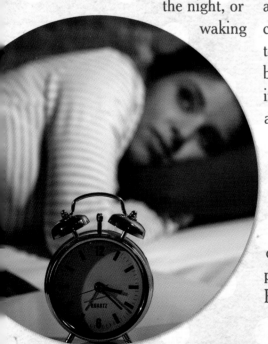

up too early. Length of sleep is not a measure of insomnia, because different people require different amounts. So, if disturbed sleep leaves you feeling fatigued and not up to par the next day, you may be suffering from insomnia, even if you slept for eight hours. Brief spells of insomnia may accompany worry, stress, changes in job shifts, or other temporary life situations. Habitual coffee drinking, even if only a few cups a day, may also cause or contribute to insomnia. Chronic insomnia may accompany such conditions as depression; chronic pain; or withdrawal from nicotine, alcohol, drugs, or sleep medications; or life passages such as menopause. Because some of these condi-

tions become more prevalent as we age, insomnia is common among the elderly.

Insomnia can be the first sign of nutritional deficiencies, appearing before more serious diseases arise. It may indicate a deficiency of the minerals calcium, magnesium, or potassium, all of which are common deficiencies in the American diet. Deficiencies of the B-vitamins (niacin, pathothenic acid, folic acid, biotin, and pyridoxine) or of vitamin E may also cause insomnia.

Chronic stress can also lead to insomnia. Our body possesses hormonal mechanisms to respond to brief periods of stress throughout the day. At night, our body is given a break from these mechanisms to recuperate. When the body adapts to persistent stress, however, we end up physically prepared to run from a bear, even at bedtime, when we should be resting. Many of the natural remedies in this section help send cues to the brain, body, and glandular system that we are safe and that it is now time to relax and recuperate in order to meet the challenges and stresses of tomorrow.

Conventional medical treatment for chronic insomnia includes drugs in the benzodiazepine class, such as Valium and Xanax. These drugs may be appropriate to induce sleep during a brief crisis, but withdrawal from them may worsen the insomnia or induce anxiety, and use for as little as six weeks may cause addiction. These drugs, as well as over-the-counter sleep medications, can also disrupt patterns of sleep, interfering

with the deepest stage of sleep known as deep delta-wave sleep. During this part of sleep, the body normally recovers from stress, rebuilds its immune system, and repairs tissues. Chronic drug use can result in a constant feeling of fatigue, however. Before you turn to prescription or over-the-counter medications, you may want to try one of the remedies below for a healthier, more natural snooze.

Water Cures for Insomniacs

Water cures were widely used to treat insomnia and many other ailments in 19th century America. Such treatments eventually became institutionalized at health spas throughout the country. In Germany and France today, these treatments are considered part of conventional medicine—a patient may receive prescriptions, paid for by insurance, to spend up to three weeks resting and receiving daily hydrotherapy sessions at a spa. Treatments for insomnia include applications of hot, cold, or neutral-temperature water. You will need to experiment to find the water temperature that helps you get to sleep, however, because different people and different types of insomnia require different treatments. In general, very hot or very cold treatments tend to stimulate rather than sedate, so it's best to use moderate temperatures.

Remedies for Insomnia

Reactive Hydrotherapy

As the name implies, hydrotherapy is therapy with water in any of its forms—ice, cold water, hot water, steam, freshwater, or water imbued with special minerals. Reactive hydrotherapy uses cool water treatments to provoke an increase in circulation in a certain area. Cold initially drives blood out of an area, but eventually the body reacts by flooding the area with blood to warm it up. In Clar-

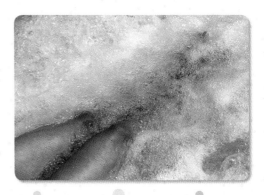

ence Meyer's *American Folk Medicine* it is noted that reactive hydrotherapy will often "Soothe the wary brain, and quiet the nerves better than an opiate." Some forms of insomnia are accompanied by excess circulation to the brain, such as might accompany mental stress. A cool compress on the neck draws blood away from the brain, helping to soothe the mind.

Directions: Put a cloth soaked in cold water on the back of the neck, and cover it with a warm towel. Keep the cloth in place for no more than fifteen minutes.

Hot Fomentation

An alternate treatment from the Seventh Day Adventists, a 150-year-old religious group that has long influenced medicine throughout North America, is to apply hot water to the back. In contrast to reactive hydrotherapy, this method uses heat to directly draw blood to the area.

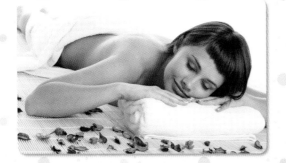

Directions: Soak a cloth in moderately hot water and rest it on the spine for twenty to thirty minutes before bedtime.

Hot Foot Bath

Another Seventh Day Adventist water treatment is the hot foot bath. The treatment draws blood away from the brain and upper body toward the feet. This is also a treatment for headaches due to congestion and menstrual cramps, so it may be especially helpful for insomnia that accompanies those conditions. You can add crushed mustard seeds to the water to increase the heating effect. Be sure to wrap the upper body in a blanket to avoid chills and promote sweating. You can also cover the head with a cloth soaked in cool water to decrease circulation to the brain. (Caution: People with insulin-dependent diabetes should not use this treatment due to the possibility of burning the feet.)

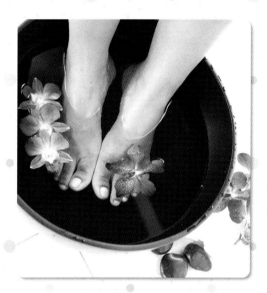

Directions: Soak the feet in hot water. The water should be moderately hot, but not so hot that you pull back from it. Continue soaking for about fifteen minutes before bedtime.

The Neutral Bath

A standard Seventh Day Adventist water treatment for insomnia and nervous exhaustion is the neutral bath. Scientific studies have shown that taking a full immersion bath quiets the production of the "fight-or-flight" hormones from the adrenal glands. Thus, this treatment is proven to relax you when you're all wound up.

Directions: Fill the tub with water at or just below body temperature, about 94–98 degrees Fahrenheit. Soak for as long as one hour before bedtime.

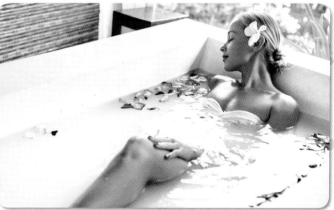

Herbal Baths

Herbal baths were popular among German immigrants, and they remain popular in Germany today. When you bathe with herbs, your skin absorbs their essential oils. An herb's aroma may also help to induce a peaceful state of mind. You can add relaxing herbs to any of the baths previously described. Avoid using oils such as peppermint, clove, and cinnamon, however. These hot oils can burn sensitive skin.

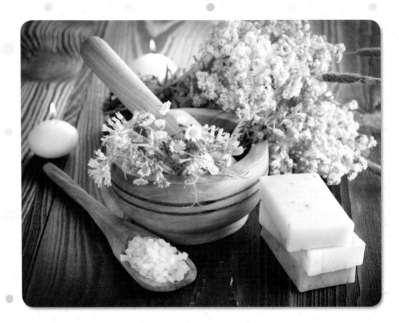

Directions: Place one ounce of valerian, hop, chamomile, or lavender in a pot and cover with a quart of boiling water. Strain and add the water to the bath. Another approach is to add two drops of essential oil to the tub water. Remember that herbal oils are highly concentrated, so a little goes a long way. Enjoy an herbal bath right before bedtime.

Dill Seeds

A natural remedy from China is to wash the head in a tea of dill seeds (*Anethum graveolens*) so you'll inhale the fumes of the tea.

Dill contains a number of sedative constituents in its volatile oil, which may explain the value of the plant for insomnia. Dill itself has not been tested by scientists for these purposes.

Directions: If you don't want to smell like a pickle all night, here's a modified version of this remedy: Put ten drops of essential oil of dill in one ounce of another oil, such as almond oil. Apply the mixture to a cloth, and keep it near your nose while you sleep. No direct application to the head is necessary. To avoid burns and blisters, never apply an essential oil in its concentrated form directly to the skin.

The Hop Pillow

A widespread cure for insomnia is the hop pillow. Hop (*Humulus lupulus*) has been used for centuries as a mild sedative. German and British immigrants, Seventh Day Adventists, Indiana farmers, and residents of the American Southwest have all used hop to help induce sleep. Hop was listed as an official medicine in the United States Pharmacopoeia from 1820 to 1926.

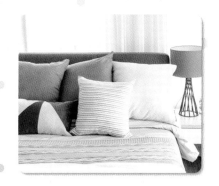

Directions: Cut two eight-by-eleven-inch squares of muslin fabric. Place one muslin square on top of the other and pin together around the edges. Sew ½-inch seams along the two long sides and one short side of the fabric, leaving the second short side open. Turn the seams to the inside. Take four ounces of hop, the fresher the better. Sprinkle it with a small amount of alcohol to bring out the active principle, but not enough to make it soggy. Add the herb to the muslin pillow case. Spread the herbs evenly within the pillow. (You will place it in your bed pillow, so you don't want it to make a lump.) Turn the raw edges under and pin the opening shut to enclose the content of the pillow securely.

Hop can also be used to make a soothing tea. Place one tablespoon of the herb in a cup and cover with boiling water. Cover the cup and let stand for ten minutes. Strain and drink before bedtime.

Rose Oil

An aromatic remedy from the Amish is to apply diluted rose oil to the forehead. The pleasant fragrance somehow tricks the brain into relaxing the body. Apply and leave on throughout the night.

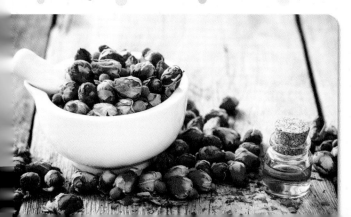

Directions: Place ten drops of concentrated rose oil in one ounce of almond oil. Apply a small amount to the forehead before going to bed.

Insomnia

Pine, Juniper, & Sage

A very common American Indian aromatherapy technique to induce sleep uses the scents of pine (*Pinus* spp.), juniper (*Juniperus* spp.), or sage (*Artemesia* spp., *Salvia* spp.). The remedy requires burning and then inhaling the fresh or dried needles or leaves of the herbs. Also, you can inhale the scent by pouring a tea made from the dried plant over hot rocks.

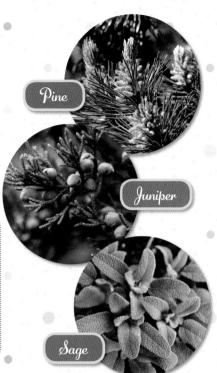

Pine

Juniper

Sage

Directions: You can adapt this technique for household use by burning the dried needles or leaves like incense. Take some dried needles or leaves of pine, juniper, or sage, light them with a match, blow the flame out, and put the smoking embers in an ashtray. Inhale the fragrance as it fills the room.

Massage

Another Seventh Day Adventist method to induce sleep is to give the person with insomnia a gentle stroking massage. Scientific research shows that massage can induce relaxation and ease stress.

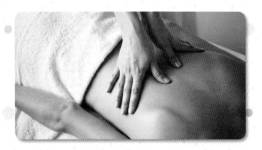

Directions: Massage the patient gently, with the strokes always moving in the direction of the heart.

Exercise

According to the Seventh Day Adventists, the best way to put yourself to sleep is to make yourself tired.

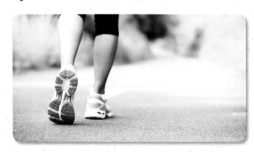

Directions: Get twenty to forty minutes of proper moderate physical exercise each day. Try going for a brisk walk or participating in a sport or a hobby you enjoy.

Deep Breathing

Another Seventh Day Adventist technique is to take slow, deep breaths. Breathing techniques are used throughout the world to relax the body and slow the mind. Research into the breathing techniques of yoga shows that deep breathing actually changes the brain waves, inducing a more relaxed state.

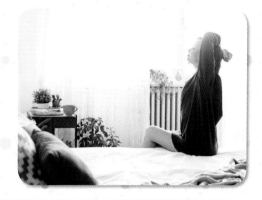

Directions: Take ten to twenty slow, deep breaths of fresh air at an open window or while lying in bed.

Passion flower

From the southern Appalachians to the American Southwest, people have long used passion flower (*Passiflora incarnata*) as a sedative to aid in sleep. The Amish combine it with chamomile. Passion flower contains sedative alkaloid constituents that help you relax.

Directions: Place a heaping teaspoon of passion flower in one cup of water and steep ten minutes. Strain and drink before retiring for the night.

Hot Milk

Drink a cup of hot milk before bed. This New England remedy has doubtlessly appeared wherever milk is consumed and persists today in the natural medicine traditions of the United States. How does it work? The warm milk may trigger instincts of safety associated with nursing at the breast. Variations of this remedy include adding ½ teaspoon of nutmeg or two teaspoons of honey. (Note: Nutmeg has psychoactive constituents that can induce unpleasant hallucinations in doses of only several teaspoons.)

Directions: Warm the milk and drink before bedtime. It'll cultivate pleasant, relaxing thoughts.

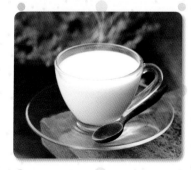

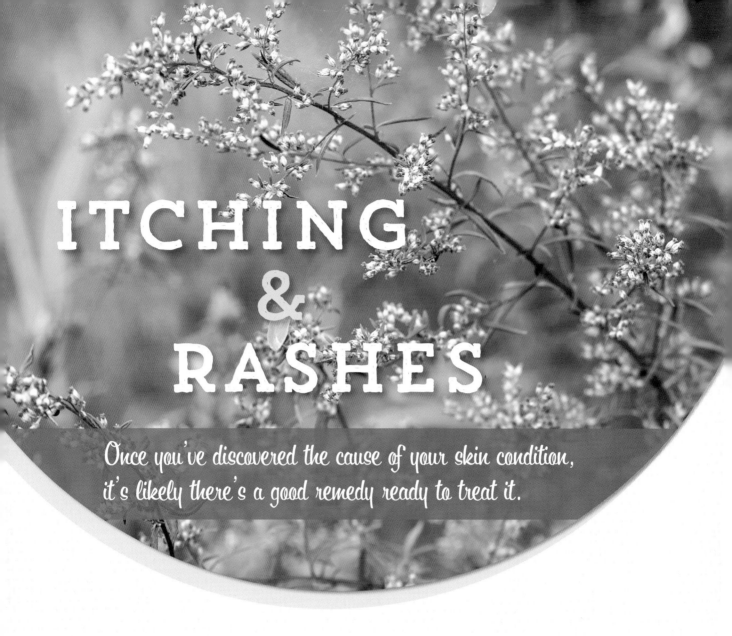

ITCHING & RASHES

Once you've discovered the cause of your skin condition, it's likely there's a good remedy ready to treat it.

An itch may be due to local irritation of the skin. Local irritation may be caused by insect bites, stings, or infestation; by an allergic reaction to a plant, animal, or synthetic substance; or by infection from molds, yeasts, or other microorganisms. Sometimes itching can be simply due to dry skin. Many prescription drugs can also cause itching.

An itch may also be due to a systemic disease—one that's irritating the skin from the inside out. For example, disorders of the blood, kidneys, or thyroid can cause itching. An itch from a systemic disease may affect only a small area of the skin, as in cases of eczema or psoriasis or allergies to substances that have been eaten. Sometimes a systemic disease will cause itching over large areas of the body or itching that moves from one place to another.

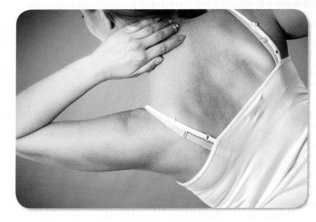

Conventional treatment of itching and rashes first requires an investigation of the cause of the skin condition. For example, if itching is the result of an allergic sensitivity to a certain fabric, avoiding that particular fabric is likely to be recommended. If prescription drugs are responsible for your discomfort, your physician may prescribe a different medication. Natural remedies traditionally rely on herbs to treat and soothe the skin. If your doctor has diagnosed your skin condition as one that can be self treated, you may want to try some of the remedies below.

Poke Root

Poke root (*Phytolacca decandra*) appears to be a universal topical remedy for itching. References to teas made from poke root that were designed to treat itching appear in American Indian lore and in the traditions of Appalachia and the South, where the plant grows. Poke root is not appropriate for internal use, however, except under medical supervision—the berries are a relatively common cause of poisoning among children.

Poke root is not usually found for sale in herb shops or health food stores. If it grows in your area, you can dig up the plant, wash and dry the roots, and chop the roots into small pieces. To make a wash, use one ounce of the root to one quart of water. Be sure to keep the plant away from children, and do not take poke root internally.

Itching & Rashes

Remedies for
ITCHING & RASHES

Juniper-Clove Salve

Folklorist Clarence Meyer's *American Folk Medicine* suggests using a salve of juniper (*Juniperus* spp.) and clove (*Eugenia caryophyllata*) to soothe itchy skin. Juniper berries have been used to treat itching by American Indians of the Paiute, Shoshone, and Cherokee tribes. Clove has been used throughout Asia, the Middle East, Mexico, and the American Southwest to treat itchy skin conditions. Juniper contains anti-inflammatory volatile substances, and clove contains the substance eugenol, a topical anesthetic widely used by dentists. The eugenol presumably affects the itch by numbing the nerve endings in the skin. The following salve is modified slightly from the one in Meyer's collection.

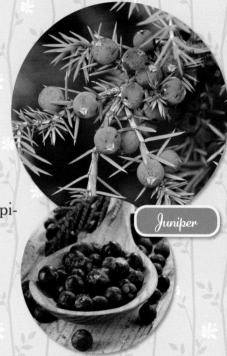

Juniper

Clove

DIRECTIONS: Melt three ounces of unsalted butter in a sauce pan. Then, in a separate pan, melt a lump of beeswax about the size of two tablespoons (it is difficult to get beeswax actually into the tablespoon). When the beeswax is melted, add it to the melted butter and stir well. Add five tablespoons of ground juniper berries and three tablespoons of ground clove to the butter/beeswax mixture and stir. (Instead of purchasing the herbs as powders, it is best to grind the herbs yourself because the volatile substances are preserved better in the whole berries and clove.) Allow the mixture to cool and become solid. Apply as a salve to itchy skin.

Basil

A wash of basil tea (*Ocimum basilicum*) is used in Chinese natural medicine to treat itching from hives. Basil, like cloves, contains high amounts of eugenol, a topical anesthetic.

DIRECTIONS: Place ½ ounce of dried basil leaves in a one-pint jar and fill with boiling water. Immediately cover to prevent the escape of the aromatic eugenol from the tea. Allow to cool to room temperature. Strain, dip a clean cloth in the tea, and apply to itchy areas as often as desired.

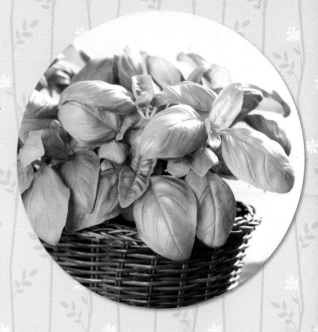

Mint

Another remedy from Chinese medicine for treating itchy skin rashes or hives is a wash of mint tea. In China, cornmint (*Mentha arvensis*) is the type of mint used. In North America, peppermint (*Mentha piperita*), which has constituents similar to cornmint, is preferred. Both peppermint and cornmint contain significant amounts of menthol, which has anesthetic and anti-inflammatory properties when applied topically. In general, mint also contains high amounts of the anti-inflammatory rosmarinic acid, which is readily absorbed into the skin.

DIRECTIONS: Place one ounce of dried peppermint leaves in a one-pint jar and fill with boiling water. Immediately cover the jar to prevent the escape of the aromatic eugenol from the tea. Allow to cool to room temperature. Strain, dip a clean cloth in the tea, and apply to the itchy area as often as necessary.

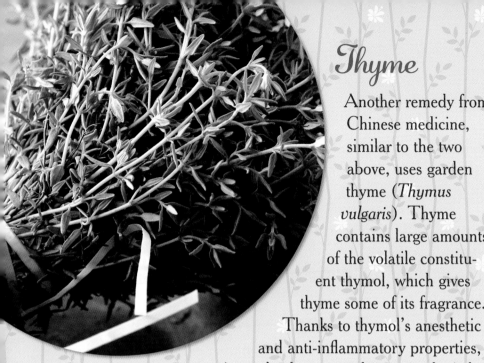

Thyme

Another remedy from Chinese medicine, similar to the two above, uses garden thyme (*Thymus vulgaris*). Thyme contains large amounts of the volatile constituent thymol, which gives thyme some of its fragrance. Thanks to thymol's anesthetic and anti-inflammatory properties, it numbs the nerves that cause the itch while reducing local inflammation. A Chinese tradition suggests mixing thyme with dandelion root.

DIRECTIONS: Place one ounce of dried dandelion root and ½ ounce of dried thyme leaves in a one-quart jar. Fill with boiling water and cover with a tight lid. Allow to cool to room temperature. Strain, dip a cloth in the tea, and apply to the affected areas.

Baking Soda Bath

A baking soda bath is recommended for itchy skin conditions in the Hispanic folklore of the Southwest. The same treatment is used in New England. Contemporary Seventh Day Adventists, a religious movement that advocates natural remedies and alternative medicine, also use baking soda baths for treating itchy skin conditions, eczema, and sunburn.

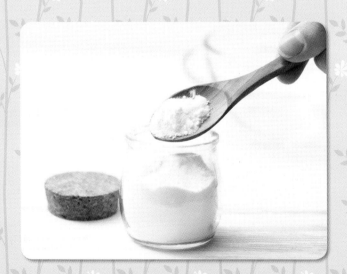

DIRECTIONS: Add one cup of commercial baking soda to a tub of 94–98 degrees Fahrenheit water. Stay in the tub for thirty to sixty minutes. Let the skin dry naturally without toweling.

Cleavers

Cleavers (*Galium aparine*) has been used to treat skin ailments since the time of the ancient Greeks. American Indians of the Iroquois and Chippewa tribes later used cleavers for the same purpose. Today, teas made from the plant remain a common prescription by professional herbalists in North America for treating skin ailments. No constituents with specific anti-inflammatory or anti-itch properties have been identified in cleavers. Herbalists theorize that the constituents work by "purifying the blood"—that is, by treating the itch from the inside out. No scientific evidence for such an action is apparent, however. Its constituents include tannins, which may account for the mild astringent action it possesses. Dried cleavers is rich in mineral nutrition, with an ounce of the herb providing significant portions of the daily requirement of such minerals as calcium, magnesium, and iron.

> **DIRECTIONS:** Place one ounce of dried cleavers in a quart of water, and simmer for twenty minutes. Strain and drink as a beverage throughout the day. Sweeten with honey if desired. Drink three cups a day for two weeks and see if your skin condition improves.

Lemon Juice

Rubbing lemon juice on itchy, inflamed skin is recommended in American folklorist Clarence Meyer's *American Folk Medicine*. The same method is used in the Hispanic folklore of the American Southwest. The aromatic substances in lemon have anesthetic and anti-inflammatory properties, which may be responsible for its medicinal activity, if any in fact exists.

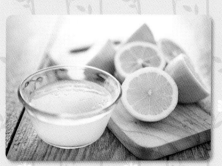

> **DIRECTIONS:** Juice a lemon. Apply undiluted to itchy skin.

MOUTH, GUMS, & TEETH

> Most oral health problems are preventable. Professional care and the prevention practices in this section are key to keeping a healthy mouth intact.

Dental problems are perhaps the oldest known conditions to afflict humanity. Prehistoric skulls from 25,000 years ago show signs of tooth decay. Remedies for tooth, mouth, and gum problems have probably existed at least since that time. By 3700 BC, the Egyptians were using tiny drills to make a hole in the jaw to drain an infected tooth. By 2700 BC, the Chinese had begun to treat tooth pain with acupuncture. The Greek physician Aesculapius introduced the pulling of diseased teeth in Greece sometime around 1200 BC. It was the barbers who pulled teeth in 17th century England.

Reliable dental anesthetics only became available in the United States during the 1800s; anesthetics were still not available in some isolated areas of this country as late as the early 1970s, however. Understandably, then, many natural remedies for toothache, mouth pain, and gum disease survive into present day in spite of more reliable professional dental care.

The best medicine for dental problems is prevention, which means regular cleaning of the teeth. Diet also has a strong impact on dental health, and, unfortunately, our modern processed foods promote tooth decay. During the 1930s, dentist and researcher Weston Price, D.D.S., visited more than 20 traditional cultures, including peoples in Europe, Africa, North and South America, Australia, and the South Sea

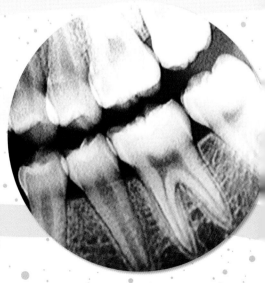

Islands. In each place, he examined the teeth of the inhabitants who ate a traditional diet and the teeth of those who ate modern foods, which were just being introduced into their villages at that time. The people eating the traditional diets averaged from one to four percent dental cavities, while those eating the modern foods averaged from twenty to forty percent. The culprits among the foods were sugar and white flour. Price photographed his research. You can see them for yourself in his book *Nutrition and Physical Degeneration*, which can still be found in print today.

The chief risk of unattended dental cavities is a dental abscess—an infection at the roots of the tooth within the jawbone. An abscess can sometimes be "silent" and cause no pain. But it may cause systemic infection and health problems far beyond the site of the infection. An abscess may require removal of the tooth. Sometimes a root canal operation is performed. In that procedure, the nerves and vascular tissue (pulp) within the tooth are removed, a disinfectant is put into the root canal, and the tooth is filled. Teeth can be "saved" in this manner and last for many decades, or even for life.

Most of the remedies in this section are for treating gum disease or sores in the mouth. If you suffer from gum disease, remember to regularly clean your teeth—you also need to floss and go for a periodic cleaning at your dentist's office. The remedies here, including the ones for dental pain, may still come in handy, though, if you are traveling in a Third World country, camping in the wilderness, or are otherwise prevented from getting immediate dental help.

Bad Breath

Many people use mouthwashes to treat bad breath, but, more often than not, the odor of bad breath is due to indigestion, not mouth infection.

If your bad breath is caused by a mouth infection, try any of the remedies in this section. Aromatics, such as clove, will also freshen the breath while disinfecting the mouth. In fact, in South Asia and the Middle East, it is a custom to chew on the seeds of aromatic spices such as clove, cardamom, or fennel after meals. These seeds contain antimicrobial substances as well as constituents that freshen the breath. Often times, the constituents that give an herb its smell and good taste are the same ones that fight infection and reduce inflammation.

Mouth, Gums, & Teeth

Remedies for the
MOUTH, GUMS, & TEETH

CLOVE

Clove (*Eugenia caryophyllata*) has been used as a toothache remedy in Asia since antiquity. Later, it moved along trade routes from Europe to the Mediterranean. By 3 BC, clove had become a universal natural remedy for dental pain in the Mediterranean. Dentists of the 19th century, in both Europe and North America, also used

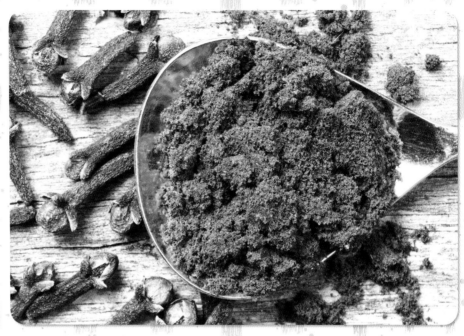

clove oil to relieve dental pain. Today, dentists use eugenol, a major ingredient in oil of clove, to relieve dental pain and to disinfect dental abscesses. Eugenol also has local anesthetic properties. Clove is still used for dental pain today in the natural medicine of New Englanders, the Amish, and Hispanics in the Southwest.

Directions: Blend up one teaspoon of clove into a powder in a coffee grinder. Moisten the powder with some olive oil and pack into a cavity or area where a filling has been lost. Alternately, you can purchase clove oil at a pharmacy or health food store. Soak a cotton ball with the oil and place on the gums next to an aching tooth. Be sure to visit your dentist promptly to prevent further tooth decay.

GOLDENSEAL

Goldenseal (*Hydrastis canadensis*) was a famous dental remedy of the early American colonists. It was used for mouth ulcers and infected gums. The related plants goldthread (*Coptis trifolia*) and Oregon grape root (*Mahonia aquifolium, Berberis aquifolium*) were used by the American Indians for the same purpose. Like goldenseal, goldthread and Oregon grape root contain the antimicrobial constituent berberine. Of the three plants, goldenseal is probably best for treating sore and swollen gums because it also contains strong astringent constituents that may help to firm up swollen gum tissues.

Directions: In a cup, pour one cup of boiling water over one teaspoon of goldenseal root. Let steep until the water reaches room temperature. Take one-ounce doses. Swish around the mouth thoroughly before swallowing. Do this three times a day as needed.

MYRRH GUM

Myrrh gum (*Commiphora myrrha*) has been used to treat mouth problems in the Middle East and North Africa since antiquity. The use of myrrh gum later spread to India, China, and Europe along Arab trade routes. Myrrh gum, like goldenseal, is astringent and tightens up loose gums. It is also antimicrobial. (The Egyptians used it in their mummification process to prevent the bacterial degradation of the corpse.) The following toothache remedy comes from an 1846 herbal tincture of the Thomsonian tradition.

Directions: Combine one and a half ounces of myrrh gum and one teaspoon of cayenne pepper in a jar containing a pint of brandy. Cover the jar, and shake it several times a day for a week. Strain and save the brandy. You now have a tincture. To treat a toothache, dip a cotton ball in the tincture and place it on the cavity. Be sure to see a dentist at the first opportunity to prevent further tooth decay.

To treat swollen and inflamed gums, make a mouthwash by combining a one-ounce shot glass of the tincture with three ounces of water. Rinse the mouth frequently during the day.

Mouth, Gums, & Teeth

WILLOW

The bark of various species of the willow tree (*Salix* spp.) have been used to treat mouth and gum infections by American Indian tribes throughout North America. Eskimo groups also used it to treat mouth infections. Although willow bark is famous for its aspirin-like constituents, it has antimicrobial constituents as well. The bark is also astringent, which can tone swollen gum tissues.

Directions: Place one ounce of willow bark in one quart of water. Bring to a boil, cover, and simmer on the lowest heat for twenty minutes. Remove from heat and let stand until the water reaches room temperature. Refrigerate and use as a mouthwash up to eight times a day.

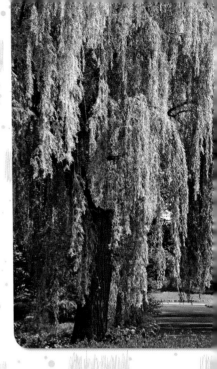

ECHINACEA

Echinacea was a universal toothache and gum disease remedy among the American Indians of the Great Plains region. Although it formerly grew in abundance in that area, echinacea is rapidly disappearing in that region due to overharvesting for worldwide medicinal use.

Applied topically, whether to skin or gums, echinacea can promote the healing of wounds and ulcers. Constituents in *Echinacea angustifolia*, the echinacea species used by the Plains Indians, are chemically related to the constituents in prickly ash that produce a tingling sensation and act as a local anesthetic. These constituents are not present in *Echinacea purpurea*, however, which is the species most often available in health food stores and herb shops, and the one most likely to be found in your garden.

Directions: Obtain a whole or chopped *Echinacea angustifolia* root at a health food store or herb shop. Grind a small amount in a coffee grinder. Pack the powder like snuff between your cheek and the tooth next to a sore area, or pack the powder directly into a cavity. Be sure to see your dentist at the first opportunity so that tooth decay does not progress.

GOLDENSEAL & MYRRH GUM

A remedy from contemporary Kentucky for sore and swollen gums calls for equal parts of goldenseal (*Hydrastis canadensis*) and myrrh gum (*Commiphora myrrha*). The combination also appears today in the natural medicine of Utah. This remedy has its roots in Thomsonian herbalism and Physiomedicalist medicine of the 19th century.

Directions: Purchase goldenseal tincture and myrrh gum tincture at a health food store or herb shop. Take one ounce of each tincture and place in an eight-ounce jar. Fill the jar with water. Cover the jar and shake well. Store the jar in the refrigerator. Use once a day as a mouthwash, or up to eight times a day for active gum disease.

YERBA MANSA

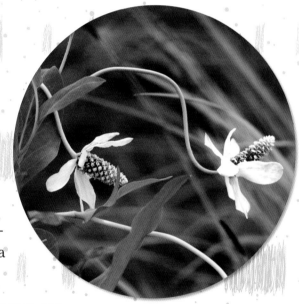

What goldenseal was to the American Indians of the eastern forests (and echinacea was to the Plains Indians), yerba mansa (*Anemopsis californica*) was to the American Southwest. All three herbs were used as panaceas for a wide variety of illnesses. Spanish settlers learned the uses of yerba mansa from the Maricopa, Pima, Tewa, and Yaqui Indian tribes. (*Yerba mansa* is short for *yerba del indio manso*, or "herb of the tamed Indians.") The Eclectic school of medicine later used yerba mansa as a mucous membrane remedy.

Directions: Place one ounce of yerba mansa in one quart of water, bring to a boil, and simmer for twenty to thirty minutes. Let stand. Refrigerate. Use as a mouthwash for gum disease or mouth sores as often as eight times a day.

Yerba mansa contains the volatile constituents thymol and methyl eugenol, both of which have demonstrated antimicrobial properties. Its other constituents, which are similar to those in goldenseal and myrrh gum, are astringent. Use yerba mansa for treating sores in the mouth.

Mouth, Gums, & Teeth

MUSCLE STRAINS & SPRAINS

Folk traditions throughout North America use irritating liniments and plasters to treat muscle injuries. For your muscle aches, try one of these "hot" remedies below.

When the body's tissues are injured, the body initiates the process of inflammation to heal them. Blood flow increases to the area, causing redness. Lymph floods the tissues, causing swelling. (The initial flooding of lymph to the area can cause severe pain as the tissues are stretched.) Chemicals that cause pain are secreted to the damaged tissues. The net effect of all this swelling and pain is to immobilize the area to prevent further injury.

Next, some of the body's white blood cells migrate to the area to clear away damaged tissue. Good circulation is necessary at this stage to bring in the nutrients necessary to build new tissue and to carry away the debris of the injury.

You can decrease the pain in the area by reducing the swelling. Soak the affected part in cool water. After the first day, however, it is important to increase circulation to the injured part. To do this, treat the area with hot soaks and massage.

Folk traditions throughout North America and other parts of the world make use of irritating liniments and plasters to treat muscle injuries. These treatments are applied externally to irritate the skin at the site of the pain—a process called counter irritation. Experiments show that counter irritation not only increases blood flow to the skin by as much as four times, but also increases blood flow and temperature to the muscles underneath the injured area. Other folk remedies for strains and sprains are taken internally and have pharmacological effects similar to aspirin.

Homeopathic Arnica

One of the most popular homeopathic remedies in United States health food stores is arnica, which is used for bruises, strains, sprains, and other painful traumas. Homeopathic remedies are highly diluted substances and are a subject of controversy in science because they often contain no traces of the original substance.

Clinical trials show that some homeopathic remedies have a medicinal effect, but conventional scientists cannot explain why they work. Homeopathic arnica supposedly will relieve traumatic pain that is accompanied by bruising and has been used this way by homeopaths for several centuries. However, at least five modern clinical trials have shown that arnica works no better than a placebo. It was tested for pain accompanying abdominal surgery, tooth extraction, and heavy exercise.

Chinese "Hit" Medicine

One branch of traditional Chinese herbal medicine, called "hit medicine," deals with the treatment of traumatic injuries. In any North American Asian market that sells herbal remedies, you can find these internal and external medicines for strains, sprains, and bruises. Liniments and plasters that stick to your skin, and other formulas, are all available. Some formulas to look for are Yunnan Pi Yao, an internal formula shown in clinical trials to reduce internal bleeding and bruising; White Flower Analgesic Balm, an external liniment; and Po Sum On medicated oil, which is also for external use.

Muscle Strains and Sprains

Remedies for
MUSCLE STRAINS & SPRAINS

Cayenne Pepper

In the folk medicine of Utah, Indiana, Illinois, Ohio, and China, cayenne pepper (*Capsicum* spp.) is used in liniments and plasters. Hispanics in the Southwest use cayenne pepper in their liniments as well. Cayenne became a popular natural remedy thanks to Thomsonian herbalism, which was a well-known herbal movement throughout rural New England and the Midwest in the early 1800s. A constituent of cayenne, called capsaicin, which is also used in police "pepper spray," stimulates pain receptors without actually burning the tissues. Thus, cayenne is one of the safest items to use for counter irritation. Below is a simple cayenne liniment.

Directions: Place one ounce of cayenne pepper in a quart of rubbing alcohol. Let the solution stand for two to three weeks, shaking the bottle each day. (You'll need to make this one in advance!) Then, apply to the affected area. (This remedy is not for internal use.)

A faster alternative is to place one ounce of cayenne pepper in one pint of boiling water. Simmer for half an hour. Do not strain, but add one pint of rubbing alcohol. Let cool to room temperature.

Probably the fastest method, from contemporary North American Chinese folklore, is to gently melt five teaspoons of Vaseline in a pan and add to it one teaspoon of cayenne pepper. Stir well and allow to cool to room temperature. Apply as desired.

Mustard Plaster

The mustard plaster, used since the dawn of history, remains today in the medical literature of Appalachia, China, and Europe. The irritating substance in mustard is not activated until the seeds are crushed and mixed with liquid.

Directions: Crush the seeds of white mustard (*Brassica alba*) or brown mustard (*Brassica juncea*) or grind them in a seed grinder. Moisten the mixture with vinegar and sprinkle with flour. Spread the mixture on a cloth. Cover with a second cloth. Lay the moist side across the   painful area. Leave on about twenty minutes. Remove if the poultice becomes uncomfortable. Wash the affected area.

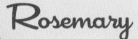

Rosemary

Rosemary (*Rosmarinus officinalis*) was used to relieve pain and spasm by doctors of the Physiomedicalist school in the last century. Today, rosemary is used (both externally and internally) in the natural medicine of Mexico and the Southwest for treating the pain of pulled muscles. Rosemary contains four anti-inflammatory substances, including rosmarinic acid, which has a biochemical action similar to aspirin. Rosmarinic acid is also easily absorbed through the skin and is approved as a topical analgesic by the German government.

Directions: Put one ounce of rosemary leaves in a one-pint canning jar and fill with boiling water. Cover tightly and let stand for thirty minutes. Apply as a wash over the painful area two to three times a day.

Each time you apply the wash, drink a 2-ounce dose of the wash as well.

Wintergreen Oil

Wintergreen (*Gaultheria procumbens*) has been used to treat muscle pain by the Delaware, Menominee, Ojibwa, Potawatomi, and Iroquois Indian tribes. It entered into official United States medicine for this purpose in 1820 and remains, in the form of wintergreen oil, a medicine included in the United States Pharmacopoeia. Wintergreen and wintergreen oil also appear as treatments for muscle pain in the natural medicine of New England.

The active pain-relieving constituent in wintergreen is methyl-salicylate, a chemical relative of aspirin. The concentrated oil has been used as a pain-relieving medicine since the 1800s, but it can be toxic, even when applied to the skin. (Aspirin was discovered during the search for safer pain-relieving drugs.) If you want to use this plant, stick with the dried herb.

Directions: Pour one pint of boiling water over one ounce of dried wintergreen leaves in a cup. Let stand until it reaches room temperature. Apply as a wash over the affected area, and, simultaneously, take two-ounce doses of the tea three to four times a day.

Witch Hazel

Witch hazel is a tree native to North America. It contains both astringent and anti-inflammatory properties. Settlers learned the use of witch hazel for treating pain from the Indians of the Oneida tribe in New York. In the 1840s, the use of the plant spread throughout the United States in the form of various over-the-counter products. The use of witch hazel later spread to Europe, where its extract became popular. Witch hazel extract remains in use today in professional British herbalism and in conventional German medicine. The German government has approved the use of witch hazel for treating minor inflammations, especially of the skin and mucous membranes. Witch hazel is also used in the natural remedy of New England as an external application for sprains.

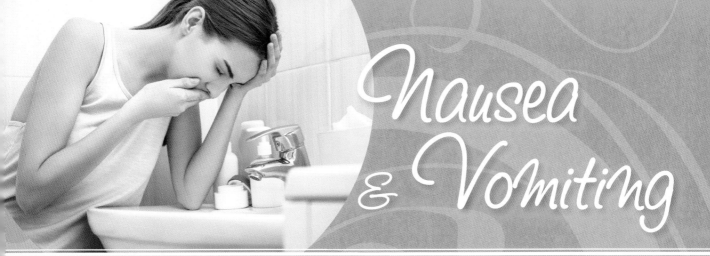

Nausea & Vomiting

Nausea and vomiting are symptoms of a wide variety of illnesses, conditions, and reactions to physical irritants. Settle your stomach with one of the remedies below.

Nausea is an extremely uncomfortable or queasy feeling in the stomach area, often accompanied by an urge to vomit. Vomiting is the forceful ejection of the contents of the stomach through the mouth.

The sensation of nausea and the urge to vomit originate in an area of the brain called the vomiting center. In response to certain messages from nerves in the digestive system or in the inner ear (part of which controls balance) or to direct stimulation by certain drugs, the vomiting center can trigger the muscular actions that result in vomiting.

Nausea most often follows food poisoning or bacterial or viral infections of the intestinal tract. The nausea center can also be stimulated by ear infections, head trauma, or other neurological conditions in the brain such as migraine headache. Poisons in the bloodstream, such as alcohol, can also trigger nausea and induce vomiting. Severe vomiting, vomiting with pain as a predominant symptom, vomiting after a head injury, or chronic nausea all require medical diagnosis and treatment. Other common causes of nausea or vomiting are prescription drugs and pregnancy.

Nausea and vomiting are usually temporary conditions that can be beneficial if they result in the expulsion of something potentially harmful to the body. However, persistent or recurring vomiting can lead to a dangerous loss of fluids and salts (called dehydration) and nutrients. This risk of dehydration is most serious in infants and the elderly, but it is also a threat in individuals with bulimia, a condition in which vomiting is induced in order to control weight gain.

Conventional treatment for simple nausea is to drink clear fluids and, if vomiting has subsided, eat dry or bland foods such as soda crackers. Pediatric electrolyte replacement fluids, available in most supermarkets and pharmacies, may be the best treatment for children and the elderly. Conventional physicians can also prescribe a variety of drugs that can successfully control the urge to vomit.

Herbal natural remedies may work in several ways. Most of the herbs are aromatic and contain volatile oils with anti-inflammatory, antispasmodic, anesthetic, and antimicrobial properties. Their ability to relieve nausea is due to the herb's gastrointestinal local "anesthetic" effect, according to R.F. Weiss, M.D., author of *Lehrbuch der Phytotherapie* (translation: *Herbal Medicine*), the standard textbook of medical herbalism used in German schools of medicine and pharmacy. When ingested, says Weiss, the herbs work by numbing the nerve endings of the stomach, thereby reducing the sensitivity of the gag reflex.

Herbs & Pregnancy

Some traditions suggest drinking coffee or black or green tea for nausea. However, all caffeine-containing drinks should be avoided during pregnancy. And, although it is still a matter of scientific debate, some trials show increased risk of miscarriage and lower birth weight for babies of mothers who consume as little as a single cup of coffee a day.

Many of the herbs in this section are contraindicated in pregnancy, especially during early pregnancy when morning sickness is most common. However, mint, ginger (doses less than five grams per day), chamomile, raspberry, and fennel are safe for use in the dosages recommended here, according to standard texts on botanical safety. The use of herbs such as catnip, cinnamon, clove, ginger (doses greater than five grams per day), thyme, and yarrow, especially in medicinal doses, should be avoided during pregnancy. Normal amounts of cinnamon, ginger, or thyme that are present in spiced foods probably present no problem, however.

Remedies for
Nausea & Vomiting

Mint

Mints such as peppermint (*Mentha piperita*) and spearmint (*Mentha spicata*) are used throughout North America and Europe for soothing nausea. The Cherokee, Micmac, and Cheyenne Indians all used mints for this purpose. Today, mints are recommended for nausea in the medical traditions of Indiana and in the Hispanic folklore of the Southwest. Mints are also used to soothe nausea in contemporary Arabic medicine.

Peppermint was used medicinally by the ancient Egyptians and was also valued by the Greeks and Romans. The 17th-century British herbalist Nicholas Culpepper wrote that "few remedies are of greater efficacy" for nausea than peppermint. Peppermint is approved in Germany as a medicine for weak digestion, and, according to a German textbook on medical herbalism, nausea is one of the top indications for using peppermint. According to the text, the plant reduces the gag reflex by anesthetizing the stomach lining.

Directions: Place one tablespoon of mint leaves in a one-pint jar and fill with boiling water. Let stand twenty to thirty minutes, shaking the bottle from time to time to mix its contents. Strain and sip as desired.

Popcorn

A nausea remedy from Indiana natural medicine calls for eating popcorn. The popcorn should be popped without oil, and then covered with boiling water. The result: a bland mush. The recommendation is consistent with the orthodox medical advice to eat bland food such as soda crackers for nausea.

Directions: Pop the popcorn in a skillet with a lid, without using oil. Place the dry popcorn in a bowl. Cover with boiling water and let stand for fifteen minutes. Eat a teaspoon of the soggy popcorn every ten minutes.

Yarrow

Yarrow (*Achillea* spp.) has been used as an antiemetic by American Indians of the Iroquois, Cheyenne, and Shoshone tribes. It is used for the same purpose in European medical traditions. Yarrow contains anti-inflammatory and anesthetic constituents. These constituents probably account for any effectiveness that the herb has for treating nausea.

Directions: Place one tablespoon of dried yarrow leaves in a one-pint jar and fill with boiling water. Cover and let stand for twenty to thirty minutes, turning or shaking the bottle from time to time. Strain and take sips of the warm tea. Don't take yarrow during pregnancy.

Ginger

Ginger (*Zingiber officinale*) is used for treating nausea in the medical traditions of New England and China. It is also approved for treating nausea by the German government. Scientific trials have shown that ginger may reduce nausea caused by several conditions, including motion sickness, morning sickness, and the nausea that accompanies chemotherapy. Doses as low as one gram have shown this effect. Ginger contains a variety of anti-inflammatory and local gastrointestinal anesthetic constituents.

Directions: Place ½ teaspoon of powdered ginger spice in a cup. Fill with boiling water. Cover and let stand for ten minutes. Strain the tea and drink in sips. Don't drink more than three cups of ginger tea per day during pregnancy. And don't drink ginger tea without consulting your doctor if you have gallstones.

German Chamomile

Chamomile tea (*Matricaria recutita*) has been used as a nausea remedy by the Cherokee Indians. It continues to be used in the traditions of New England. Chamomile contains powerful anti-inflammatory and analgesic substances that may reduce the gag reflex. Chamomile is approved as a digestive remedy by the German government, although not specifically for nausea.

Directions: Place two tablespoons of chamomile flowers in a one-pint jar and fill with boiling water. Let stand twenty to thirty minutes, shaking the bottle from time to time to mix its contents. Strain and sip as desired.

Peppermint

An antinausea formula found in the folk traditions of the Kentucky Appalachian mountains is a combination of peppermint and chamomile. The two herbs are more often used together than separately.

Directions: Place one tablespoon each of chamomile flowers and peppermint leaves in a one-pint jar and fill with boiling water. Let stand twenty to thirty minutes, shaking the bottle from time to time to mix its contents. Strain and sip as desired.

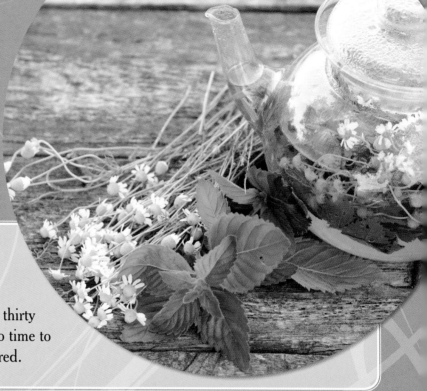

Raspberry Leaf Tea

The Amish suggest a tea of raspberry leaves (*Rubus idaeus*) for treating nausea. The Thompson and Kwakiutl Indians used the leaves of related members of the *Rubus* genus in the same manner. No specific antinauseant or anesthetic properties have been identified in raspberry leaf constituents, but the tannin constituents in the leaves may have an anti-inflammatory or soothing effect on the digestive tract wall.

Directions: Place one ounce of raspberry leaves in a one-quart jar. Fill with boiling water. Place a lid on the jar and let the tea stand until it reaches room temperature. Shake the bottle from time to time to mix its contents. Drink freely.

Electrolyte Replacement Therapy

The main health hazard of excessive vomiting is dehydration and the loss of electrolyte salts. Replacement drinks are available in supermarkets and pharmacies, or you can make your own. The World Health Organization formula for an electrolyte replacement beverage after excessive diarrhea or vomiting is:

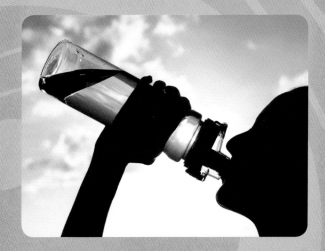

- Three and a half grams sodium chloride (table salt)
- Two and a half grams sodium bicarbonate (baking soda)
- One and a half grams potassium chloride (obtained at pharmacy)
- Twenty grams of glucose (also obtained at pharmacy)
- One liter of water (One quart and two ounces)

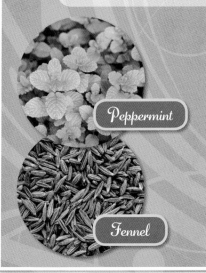

Peppermint

Fennel

A German medical text suggests the following formula, which includes peppermint (*Mentha piperita*) and fennel (*Foeniculum vulgare*), two herbs often used in treating nausea: Make a tea by simmering one tablespoon each of peppermint leaves and fennel seed in one quart of water for fifteen minutes in a covered pot. Strain and allow to cool to room temperature. To this add ½ teaspoon salt, ¼ teaspoon of baking soda, ¼ teaspoon potassium chloride, and two tablespoons of glucose. Drink freely.

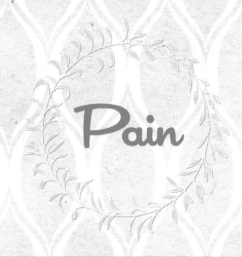

Pain

Pain is a signal—it is often a sign of disease, injury, or abnormal changes in the body.

Pain is an unpleasant or uncomfortable sensation that can range from mild irritation to excruciating agony. It is probably the most commonly reported symptom and is linked to innumerable disorders and diseases.

Pain occurs when specialized nerve endings are stimulated; within a fraction of a second this pain "signal" travels through a network of nerves to the brain. Pain can be a warning sign, indicating impending damage to the body, or it can be a protective mechanism, causing the person feeling pain to remove the cause or reflexively draw away from the source.

Most healthy people have occasional, brief twinges of pain that have no specific cause and are usually harmless. However, bothersome, recurring, or persistent pain can be caused by thousands of factors. Most commonly, pain is a symptom of disease, injury, or abnormal changes in the body.

There are many types of pain. Pain can be dull and constant, sharp and sudden, crushing, burning, piercing, or aching. When it is felt in areas other than the location of the disorder (for example, when the pain of heart attack is felt in the arm), it is called referred pain. Unexplainable pain should be reported promptly to a doctor for investigation to locate its source for it to be treatment.

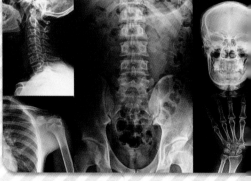

Using plants to quiet pain goes back before the dawn of recorded medical history, but none of these plants proved particularly effective. That is why this century brought about newer and better pain drugs and why pain medications are among the most popular over-the-counter drugs. Many of the modern drugs, such as aspirin, acetaminophen, ibuprofen, and corticosteroids, suppress the formation of prostaglandins, a class of chemicals in the local tissues that trigger pain. There are other, more potent painkillers, such as the opiates, morphine, and codeine, but these must be prescribed by a doctor.

Many of the plants used in natural medicine for pain relief use the same biochemical pathways as the non-opiate pain-relieving drugs, but they are not as effective. On the other hand, many of these plants have multiple effects. Their antispasmodic and circulation-promoting constituents may make up for what these plants lack in prostaglandin-suppressing strength. Comparative trials of these plants with drugs have not been performed, but the plants' persistent use in natural medicine (even with the availability of inexpensive over-the-counter drugs) indicates that they must have at least some beneficial effect. Herbal formulas that combine prostaglandin-suppressing, antispasmodic, sedative, and antidepressant plants are commonly prescribed by professional herbalists in North America, Great Britain, and Australia (see sidebar, "Formulas for Chronic Pain").

Traditions throughout North America and other parts of the world also make use of irritating liniments and plasters to treat muscle and joint pain. These natural remedies are applied externally to irritate the skin over the site of the pain. Physiological tests show that such treatments increase blood flow to the skin by as much as four times and also increase blood flow and temperature in the muscles underneath the skin. Any relief from such treatments is due to this increased circulation to the area, which ensures a healthy flow of oxygen to the tissues and relieves the swelling of stagnant lymph in the area. This method, called counterirritation, may also increase local or systemic levels of endorphins, the body's natural pain-killing substances that are more potent than opiates.

Formulas for Chronic Pain

Although acute pain may be best treated with pharmaceutical drugs, medical herbalists of countries such as Great Britain, North America, Australia, and New Zealand often use combinations of herbs and hydrotherapy to treat chronic pain. Chronic pain often creates a constellation of problems—besides the pain itself, tension, spasm, insomnia, or depression can often result. And while conventional pain medications may remedy one or two of these side effects, some formulas of herbs can address them all. A pain-reliever, an antispasmodic, a sedative, and an antidepressant may all be in included in a typical herbal formula created by a medical herbalist. For example, one herbal combination may include equal parts of willow bark (for pain), cramp bark (for spasm), valerian (a sedative), and St. John's wort (an antidepressant).

Remedies for Pain

Hot Peppers

Cayenne pepper (*Capsicum* spp.) is used in formulas for liniments and plasters in the natural medicine of China, the American Southwest, Utah, and throughout Ohio, Indiana, and Illinois. External and internal use of cayenne pepper to stimulate circulation was a key element of Thomsonian herbalism throughout rural New England and the Midwest in the early 1800s. (The Thomsonian movement of herbalism was introduced into practice in the early 19th century by Samuel Thomson, an influential New England herbalist. Thomsonian herbalism has been a powerful influence on American herbal traditions for the last 190 years.) Capsaicin, a constituent of cayenne, stimulates pain receptors without actually burning the tissues. Cayenne is thus one of the safest items to use for counterirritation. Below is a simple cayenne liniment.

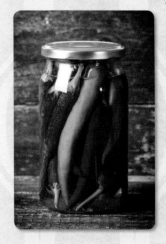

Directions: Place one ounce of cayenne pepper in a quart of rubbing alcohol. Let the mixture stand for three weeks, shaking the bottle each day. Then, apply to the affected part during acute attacks.

Alternately, if you can't wait three weeks for relief, try this method: Place one ounce of cayenne pepper in a pint of boiling water. Simmer for half an hour. Do not strain, but add a pint of rubbing alcohol. Let cool to room temperature. Apply as desired to the affected part. (Do not ingest either of these remedies.)

Cramp Bark & Black Haw

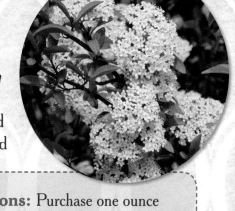

For the treatment of spasmodic pain, both cramp bark (*Viburnum opulus*) and black haw (*Viburnum prunifolium*) have been used in American Indian medicine. The Cherokee, Delaware, Fox, and Ojibwa tribes all used cramp bark to treat both menstrual pain and muscle spasm. Cramp bark and black haw were used for arthritic or menstrual pain in Physiomedicalist and Eclectic medicine. The plants contain the antispasmodic and muscle-relaxing compounds esculetin and scopoletin. The antispasmodic constituents are best extracted with alcohol (rather than water), so tinctures may be more effective than teas. Black haw also contains aspirin-like compounds.

Directions: Purchase one ounce each of cramp bark and black haw tincture in a health food store or herb shop. If both aren't available, either one will do. Mix them together, and take two droppers every two or three hours for up to three days.

Willow Bark

Willow bark (*Salix alba*) was used for treating pain by the ancient Greeks more than 2,400 years ago. American Indians throughout North America, from the Houma in Louisiana and Alabama to the Ninivak Eskimos in the Arctic, used it as a pain reliever even before the arrival of the European colonists. Investigation of salicin, a pain-relieving constituent in willow bark, led to the discovery of aspirin in 1899. Although aspirin is now the top-selling pain-relieving drug in the world, willow bark is still used for treating pain in the medicine of Indiana, New England, and the Southwest, as well as by professional medical herbalists throughout the English-speaking world. The German government has approved the use of willow bark by conventional physicians for pain and fever. The most important active constituent is salicin, but other anti-inflammatory constituents also appear in the willow bark.

Directions: Purchase willow bark capsules in a health food store or herb shop. Take as directed on the label. Also, you can place two teaspoons of powdered willow bark in a cup, fill with boiling water, and let steep for fifteen to twenty minutes. Sweeten with honey if desired, and drink up to four cups a day for five to seven days, as desired.

Pain

Ginger

Ginger is used to treat various sorts of pain in the medicine of China. It is also used for pain or spasm in the medicine of New England, Appalachia, North Carolina, and Indiana. It is an important pain medication in contemporary Arabic medicine; reports of its use there in treating migraine headache and arthritis show its effectiveness. Ginger contains twelve different aromatic anti-inflammatory compounds, including some with mild aspirin-like effects.

Directions: Cut a fresh ginger root (about the size of your thumb) into thin slices. Place the slices in a quart of water. Bring to a boil, and then simmer on the lowest possible heat for thirty minutes in a covered pot. Let cool for thirty more minutes. Strain and drink one cup, sweetened with honey, as desired.

Rosemary

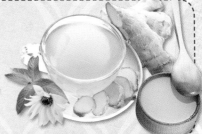

Drinking rosemary tea for pain is a remedy used in the contemporary Hispanic medicine of Mexico and the Southwest. Rosemary has not been tested in clinical trials, but it was used to relieve pain and spasm by doctors of the Physiomedicalist school in the last century. Its leaf also contains four anti-inflammatory substances—carnosol, oleanolic acid, rosmarinic acid, and ursolic acid. Carnosol acts on the same anti-inflammatory pathways as both steroids and aspirin; rosmarinic acid acts through at least two separate anti-inflammatory biochemical pathways; and ursolic acid, which makes up about four percent of the plant by weight, has been shown in animal trials to have anti-arthritic effects.

Directions: Put ½ ounce of rosemary leaves in a one-quart canning jar and fill the jar with boiling water. Cover tightly and let stand for thirty minutes. Drink a cup as hot as possible before going to bed, and have another cupful in the morning before breakfast.

Epsom Salt Baths

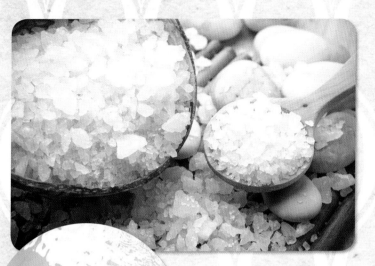

Traditions in both New England and Indiana call for Epsom salt baths to relieve pain. Epsom salt was named after a salt found in abundance in spring water near the town of Epsom, England, in 1618. The salt was reputed to have magical healing properties. Epsom salt is now produced industrially and not from the springs in England. Epsom salt is primarily magnesium sulfate and has been used medicinally in Europe for more than three hundred years. The heat of an Epsom salt bath can increase circulation and reduce the swelling of arthritis, and the magnesium can be absorbed through the skin. Magnesium is one of the most important minerals in the body, participating in at least 300 enzyme systems. Magnesium has both anti-inflammatory and anti-arthritic properties.

Hydrotherapy for Pain

During the 19th century in the United States, hydrotherapy was a popular form of medical treatment, especially for pain. The practice survives today mainly in the Appalachians and among the Seventh Day Adventists. (Hydrotherapy is also taught in naturopathic medical schools.)

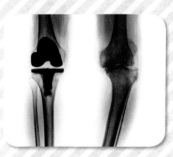

Cold water or ice is recommended for acute pain; the cold suppresses inflammation and swelling. Hot water or alternating hot and cold water (ending with cold) is the prescription for chronic pain. Hot water or alternating hot and cold water increases local circulation and has the same benefits as counterirritation. Also, research shows that full body immersion (up to the neck) reduces swelling in inflamed joints.

Homeopathic Remedies

Homeopathic medicine is based on the principle of similars, the idea that "like cures like." Homeopathic medicine holds that a substance that causes certain symptoms when given in large doses to a healthy person can cure an ill person with the same symptoms when given in very small doses. This idea that the same substance that can cause symptoms can also be used to heal is often met with skepticism.

Homeopathic remedies are highly diluted substances and are thus a subject of controversy in science. In fact, some are so diluted that they contain no traces of the original substance. Although clinical trials have shown that some homeopathic remedies do have a medicinal effect, conventional scientists have yet to prove how they work.

Perhaps the most popular homeopathic remedy sold in United States health food stores for treating pain is arnica, though it has not withstood the validity tests of clinical trials. Undiluted arnica contains various anti-inflammatory and wound-healing substances and has been used as a pain medication in the past. Users of homeopathic arnica claim the herb relieves traumatic pain that is accompanied by bruising. However, at least five clinical trials have shown that it works no better than a placebo. It was tested for the pain accompanying abdominal surgery, tooth extraction, and heavy exercise. Tests of homeopathic arnica for surgical or dental trauma have also shown the herb to be no better than a placebo for treating pain from those conditions.

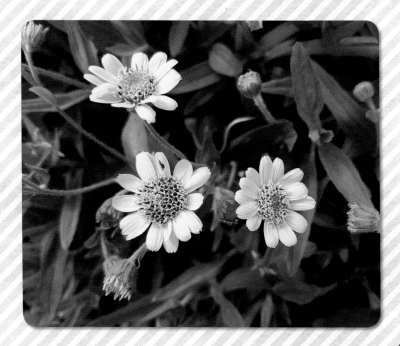

POISON IVY & OAK

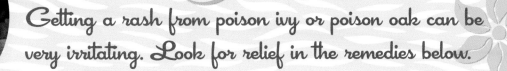

Poison oak

Getting a rash from poison ivy or poison oak can be very irritating. Look for relief in the remedies below.

A rash from poison ivy or poison oak is caused by an allergic reaction to the oil, or sap, found inside the plant. This oil, which is clear to slightly yellow, is called urushiol. It oozes from any crushed or cut part of the leaves and stem, so just brushing against a plant may not elicit a reaction. Oil content in the plants runs highest in the spring and summer, but cases are reported even in the winter.

The first exposure to the plant does not usually cause a reaction, but it does start the process of preparing the immune system to react to subsequent exposures. That preparation can take two weeks or more, and during that time, you may seem to be immune to the plants' poisons. Once the sensitization of the immune system is complete, however, severe rashes may occur. This sudden appearance of sensitivity to the plants, after seeming immunity, can be confusing to victims, but it is the result of the normal processes of the immune system. Further adding to the confusion, urushiol is actually a mixture of related compounds, and it may be more or less allergenic depending on the mix, which may vary from plant to plant, climate to climate, and season to season. Urushiol is a resinous substance that can survive burning of its plant host, so beware of smoke from weed-burning fires, which can transport the poisonous resin in the smoke.

Common anti-allergic drugs such as antihistamines are ineffective against the type of allergic reaction these plants cause. Instead, steroid drug administration is the conventional treatment. Another important treatment for urushiol allergy is a thorough washing of the affected area with soap and water to remove the poison from the skin.

The natural remedies in this section fall into three categories: Some are astringent, which helps reduce the swelling of the allergic rashes. Some have anti-inflammatory properties that work similarly to steroid drugs. And some work by washing the plant poisons from the skin.

Trying Astringents

Probably the most famous over-the-counter treatment for poison ivy or poison oak in North America is calamine lotion, which is composed of zinc oxide. (*Calamine* is a term of the medieval alchemists for zinc oxide; the word is derived from the older Latin and Greek words for zinc.) Calamine lotion acts as a drying astringent to reduce the swelling of the rash. It is also slightly disinfectant. There are several remedies in this section that also have astringent properties, including coffee, gumweed, clay, and charcoal.

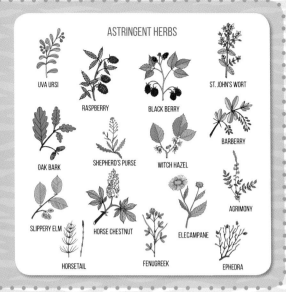

ASTRINGENT HERBS

UVA URSI
RASPBERRY
BLACK BERRY
ST. JOHN'S WORT
OAK BARK
SHEPHERD'S PURSE
WITCH HAZEL
BARBERRY
SLIPPERY ELM
HORSE CHESTNUT
ELECAMPANE
AGRIMONY
HORSETAIL
FENUGREEK
EPHEDRA

Digesting Poison

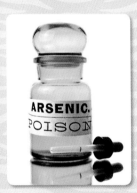

Natural medicine tradition shows an awareness of the idea that tolerance to poisons is increased by exposure. This is true of a great many toxic substances, from alcohol to arsenic. Based on this notion, which has a superficial similarity to the medical idea of allergic desensitization, there is a wide-spread claim that eating small amounts of poison ivy will gradually produce immunity. This is a very dangerous practice, though, because certain individuals could develop life-threatening reactions.

Eating Poison

In both North Carolina and Indiana, it is believed that eating poison ivy leaves prevents contraction of the poison ivy rash. And although the mucous membranes of the mouth and digestive tract would not produce the same kind of allergic reactions that cause the rash, this is still a risky practice. Certain sensitive individuals could have other, severe reactions. Carelessness while eating the leaves could also result in a poison ivy rash on the hands or lips. In sensitive individuals, life-threatening allergic shock could occur.

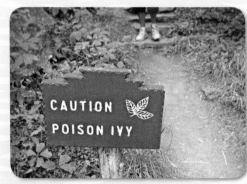

Poison Ivy

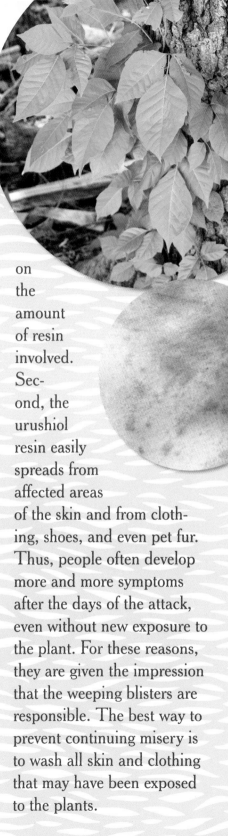

The rash and blisters that result from contact with either poison ivy or poison sumac are caused by a plant resin called urushiol. For those who are sensitive to urushiol, contact with these plants can be a source of great misery, and, along with those terribly itchy blisters, severe cases can bring on headache and fatigue. As is true of many sensitivities, reaction to urushiol can change (increase or decrease) over time and with exposure.

Poison ivy remedies, unlike any other set of cures, are practically never magical. Instead they employ herbs and common household substances such as soap and vinegar. Many of these remedies are effective, at least for symptomatic relief, though most have never been scientifically studied. A well-known treatment and preventive involves washing with old fashioned, brown laundry soap. (Actually, because urushiol is soluble in water, washing promptly with anything that includes water will help.) Another recommended wash is bleach mixed with horse urine, but soap and water are just as effective.

Prevention, of course, is better than treatment, and natural remedies offer plenty of ideas. In the Ozarks, it is said that large doses of sulfur and molasses, with a pinch of saltpeter (sodium nitrate), taken for a few weeks will confer immunity. A tea made from jewelweed is commonly applied to poison ivy rashes, but it is also said to give immunity if consumed regularly throughout the spring and summer months.

Tradition states that the poison ivy rash is spread by the contents of the blisters. This is not true, however, since the liquid in the poison ivy blister is the same liquid found in any blister. The idea originated from two facts. First, symptoms of poison ivy can appear hours to days after exposure, partly depending on the amount of resin involved. Second, the urushiol resin easily spreads from affected areas of the skin and from clothing, shoes, and even pet fur. Thus, people often develop more and more symptoms after the days of the attack, even without new exposure to the plant. For these reasons, they are given the impression that the weeping blisters are responsible. The best way to prevent continuing misery is to wash all skin and clothing that may have been exposed to the plants.

Poison Ivy & Oak

Remedies for
POISON IVY & OAK

Vinegar Wash

A vinegar wash to relieve the rash of poison ivy is reported in the folklore of Indiana and also in the southern Appalachian mountains. Vinegar washes are popular in many areas of the country for treating itching from various causes, including insect bites and allergic rashes. No scientific reason for the reduction of itching is apparent. It is recommended that the affected area is first washed with soap. Washing with soap and then vinegar may help to completely remove any plant poison from the skin.

Directions: Wash the affected area well with soap and water. Then apply vinegar, scrub lightly, and rinse.

Gumweed

Gumweed (*Grindelia camporum, Grindelia squarrosa*), a species of *grindelia*, is an American Indian remedy that was eventually adopted by the medical profession as a treatment for rashes caused by poison ivy and poison oak. Native to the American Southwest and Mexico, the gumweed plant was used as a cough medicine and treatment of skin afflictions—including poison oak—by Indians in those areas. Its use entered into the medicine of nearby colonists and settlers, and, in the last century, it was adopted into use by conventional physicians. Gumweed was an official medicine in the United States Pharmacopoeia from 1882 until 1926. It remains an official remedy in German medicine—it is used as an expectorant for coughs. The resin contains anti-inflammatory and expectorant constituents.

Directions: Apply the sticky sap from the leaves or flowers of gumweed to the affected areas. Reapply every few hours. Alternately, you can purchase tincture of *grindelia* and use it as a wash. Reapply the wash every few hours as well.

Jewelweed

Jewelweed (*Impatiens pallida, Impatiens fulva, Impatiens biflora*) is probably the most famous of the natural remedies for treating rashes caused by poison ivy. Jewelweed grows in the same sort of soil and climates as poison ivy, and can often be located near poison ivy in the eastern parts of the United States. Also called "touch-me-not," jewelweed is native to North America. It was a common remedy for poison ivy rash among the eastern American Indians, including the Cherokee and Iroquois. The Indians taught the colonists how to use jewelweed. Its use persists today in the medicine of New England, and the Appalachians.

The physicians of the Eclectic and Physiomedicalist schools of the 19th and early 20th centuries also used jewelweed as a poison ivy remedy and anti-inflammatory treatment for other allergic swellings of the skin. A report in the *Physio-Medicalist Dispensatory*, a medical text published by Dr. William Cook , M.D., in 1869, relates a medical case in which jewelweed sap was spread on the severely swollen leg of a young man bitten by a snake. Although the man's life had been at risk, his recovery began immediately after the jewelweed was applied. Thirty years later, Eclectic physicians were using poultices of the plant that were boiled in milk to treat skin conditions. *The King's American Dispensatory*, an Eclectic text from 1898, stated that when the juice of the plant is applied to poison ivy, it "gives prompt relief." Dr. Harvey Felter's *The Eclectic Materia Medica, Pharmacology, and Therapeutics* (1922) states that, when jewelweed is applied to poison ivy, "The relief is almost magical." Felter, a leading Eclectic educator, was a conservative physician best known for removing many ineffectual herbal remedies from Eclectic use. Thus, his positive statement about jewelweed was all the more significant and influential.

Modern scientific testing of jewelweed has yielded mixed results. A 1950 study found jewelweed to be of no medicinal value. Another study in 1957 found that 108 of 115 patients were completely relieved of their rash symptoms in two to three days. A 1997 study found jewelweed to be of no value in preventing poison ivy. These variable results may be due to the experiments' designs. The traditional use is to place the sap from a fresh-picked plant directly on the blisters as soon as they appear. This method was not followed in the 1997 study, but, instead, an unspecified extract of the plant was applied to artificially produced poison ivy.

Directions: At the first appearance of poison ivy rash or poison oak blisters, pick some jewelweed. Crush the plant and apply the juicy sap directly to the poison ivy rash. Alternately, you can cut the plant a few inches above the ground and slit the stem lengthwise with a knife. This may expose the juicy sap more efficiently than when crushing the plant. Leave the juice in place for several hours. Reapply continuously for several days.

Poison Ivy & Oak

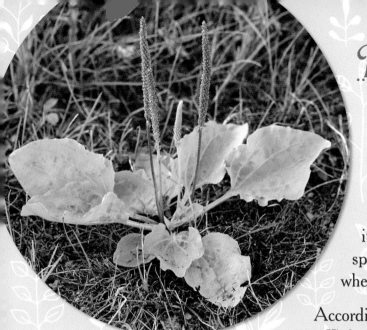

Plantain

Plantain leaf (*Plantago major*), used either as a wash or a poultice, is used to treat poison ivy in the medicine of New England and the southern Appalachians. Plantain's common names include "White Man's Footprint" and "Englishman's Footprint," names that reflect its arrival on the continent with the English-speaking immigrants and its subsequent spread wherever they moved.

According to *Herbal Medicine Past and Present (Volume II)*, by John K. Crellin and Jane Philpott, Tommie Bass, a folk herbalist from northern Georgia, recommends making a tea of plantain leaf for treating the poison ivy rash. The leaf can be boiled in either water or milk and then used as a wash on the affected part. New England folklore calls for shredding the leaves, crushing them until they become juicy with plant sap, and then applying the crushed leaves to the skin.

Plantain, which is used throughout North America as a remedy for various skin inflammations and infections, contains several different anti-inflammatory compounds, including caffeic acid, chlorogenic acid, cinnamic acid, and p-coumaric acid. In laboratory trials, these four compounds act to inhibit an enzyme in the cells called lipoxygenase. Corticosteroid drugs also inhibit this enzyme, giving these drugs their anti-inflammatory effects. Plantain itself has not been tested in clinical trials, but these and its other anti-inflammatory compounds may account for the plant's effectiveness in suppressing the inflammation caused by poison ivy or poison oak.

Directions: Pick some fresh plantain leaves. (Dried leaves probably won't work.) Shred them with your fingers, crush them until they become juicy, and press them into a poultice. Cover the affected area with the poultice and wrap with a bandage for twenty-four hours to hold the poultice in place.

Milkweed Sap

A remedy from Indiana folklore is to squeeze the milky sap of milkweed (*Asclepias syriaca*) on the poison ivy rash. Milkweed was used by American Indians for various skin conditions, including warts and bee stings, but not specifically for poison ivy or poison oak.

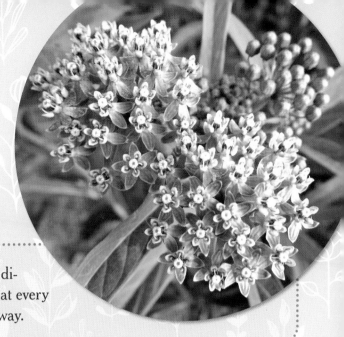

Directions: Squeeze the milky juice of milkweed directly onto the area affected by the poison ivy. Repeat every few hours until itching subsides and the rash goes away.

Aloe Vera

Aloe vera, more famously known for treating burns, may also be helpful for treating rashes caused by poison ivy or poison oak, according to the traditions of the Seventh Day Adventists. Aloe vera's anti-inflammatory constituents, which reduce blistering and inflammation in burns, may also reduce the inflammation of the skin caused by the plant poisons.

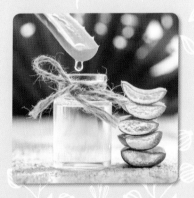

Directions: Break off a piece of a leaf of an aloe vera plant. Apply the juicy sap to the affected itchy area. (For a large area, juice some leaves in a juicer and spread the juice over the skin.) Allow the sap to dry. Gently wash off the sap and reapply every two hours. Alternately, you can purchase aloe vera gel at a health food store.

Coffee

According to *Herbal Medicine Past and Present (Volume II)*, by John K. Crellin and Jane Philpott, Appalachian folk herbalist Tommie Bass suggests washing a poison ivy rash with black coffee. Coffee beans contain five to ten percent chlorogenic acid, an anti-inflammatory constituent that acts in the same way as steroid drugs. Neither coffee nor chlorogenic acid has been tested as a treatment for poison ivy or poison oak.

Directions: Brew a pot of strong black coffee. Allow it to cool to a tolerable temperature. Use it to wash the affected area as often as desired.

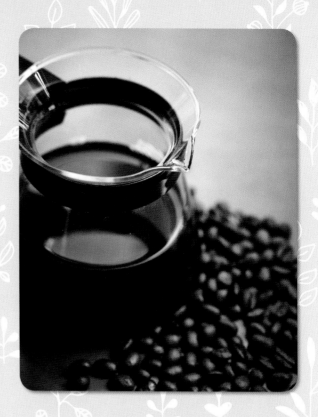

Clay Applications

Physicians of the Seventh Day Adventist tradition use clay packs to treat rashes from poison ivy or poison oak. (The same method is widespread throughout the world for treating various types of skin conditions.) Clay binds to different types of poisons; thus, it may bind to the poison ivy resins in a similar manner and remove them from the skin. And, even after the clay has been applied to the skin and the resin has been removed, the clay continues to work, helping to relieve itching. In conventional medicine, clay is sometimes used internally as a treatment for some types of poisoning.

Directions: Mix bentonite clay or cosmetic grade clay with water to make a thin paste. Paint this onto the affected area. Let the clay dry. Flake the dry clay off the skin and dispose of it in a wastebasket. (Do not put the clay down your drain because it can clog the pipes.) Reapply as often as desired.

Charcoal

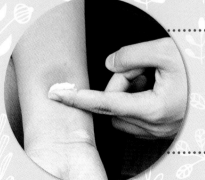

A charcoal poultice is a medical treatment of the Seventh Day Adventists for treating rashes resulting from poison ivy and poison oak. Charcoal has powerful drying and drawing properties and may help to remove any of the plant poison still on the skin.

Directions: Grind up three tablespoons of flaxseed in a coffee grinder or blender. Mix with an equal amount of crushed charcoal. (The oily flaxseed acts to hold the mixture together.) Let stand for ten to thirty minutes, mixing occasionally. Apply to the affected area and secure with a bandage. Leave in place for six to ten hours. Remove and wash the area with a cold cloth. Repeat every day until the rash is gone.

Baking Soda

Baking soda, either made into a paste or directly added to bathwater, is a poison ivy remedy from New England and Indiana. Physicians of the Seventh Day Adventist tradition also recommend the baking soda bath. This method, which cures all types of itching, appears throughout North American medicine, although no scientific reason for its effectiveness is evident. A thick paste of baking soda applied to skin affected by poison ivy or poison oak may remove any traces of the plant poison.

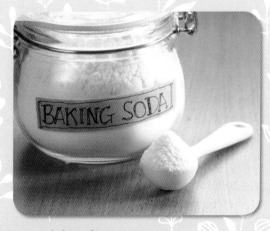

Directions: Make a paste of baking soda and apply it to the affected areas. Change the application every two hours, for a total of three applications each day. Then take a baking soda bath each day until the rash is gone.

Poison Ivy & Oak

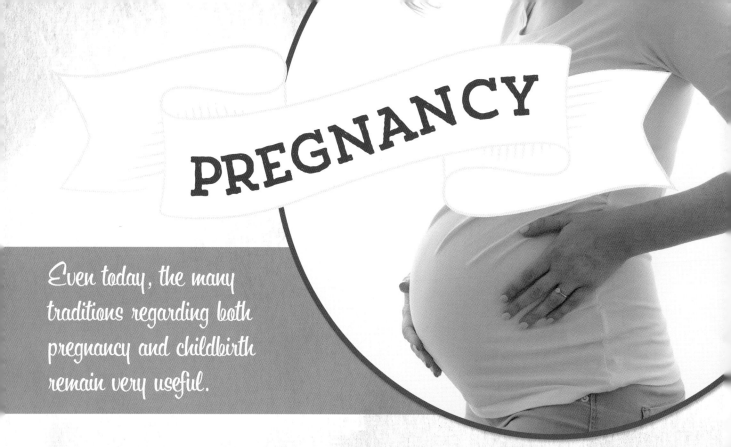

PREGNANCY

Even today, the many traditions regarding both pregnancy and childbirth remain very useful.

Until the 20th century, almost every birth in North America was a home birth, and most of these births were attended by midwives or folk healers rather than physicians. Because of this, there are many traditions regarding both pregnancy and childbirth. But most of these remedies are no longer appropriate in our modern society. Because of the risks inherent in childbirth, many women died giving birth in the era when natural remedies were the only assistance available. Maternal death was greatly reduced with the introduction of hospital births. Even home birth is safer today, because midwives are trained to screen for problem pregnancies and to transfer the mother to a hospital if complications develop. Midwives may still use some remedies, and they may work, but individuals should not try using them on their own. Some remedies that traditionally are used to "prepare for childbirth" and are given to the mother in the last month of pregnancy can actually cause prolonged labor or cause more painful contractions if taken incorrectly.

The herbs in this section fall into two categories: mineral-rich nourishing herbs and plants that help with morning sickness. Follow your doctor's or midwife's advice if you want to try these remedies.

HERBS IN PREGNANCY

The guiding principle for taking herbs during pregnancy is not to take any substance that could cause miscarriage or harm the fetus. Although no accidental miscarriages due to the use of herbs or natural remedies appear in the scientific literature, prudent advice is to avoid the use of herbs that traditionally have been used to induce abortion or to promote menstruation.

Many herbs that are normally beneficial to women should also be avoided during pregnancy. These include stimulating laxatives and some popular herbs that contain steroidal or alkaloid components (such as comfrey leaf, coltsfoot, goldenseal, dong quai, ginseng, and hop). In general, the rule is not to take any herb unless you know it is regarded as safe. The herbs in this section have all been classified as safe in pregnancy in the *Botanical Safety Handbook*, published by the American Herbal Products Association, which reviews the world's literature on herbal safety and contraindications.

PREDICTING BABY

Once a child in conceived, there is usually much speculation about its gender. Divination rituals such as a thread-and-needle pendulum over the mother's belly (which is believed to move in a circle for a girl or a straight line for a boy) are standard baby shower games. Physical signs noted in the mother are also considered—whether she "carries" high or low, whether her stomach is round or pointed, whether she is big or small, and so on.

Ideas about the baby's gender are often linked to the circumstances of its conception. For example, if the father's desire for a child was strongest, it would be a boy; if the mother's desire was great, a girl. Conception just before menstruation could result in a boy; just after, a girl. An ax placed under the bed could lead to a boy; scissors were used in hopes for a girl. If the weather was dry, look for a boy; if it was rainy, it might be a girl. As is typical in folk tradition, these elements are often reversed in differing cultures. There is one exception to this reversal, however: There's a notion that claims a woman is prettier when she is carrying a boy—because she has to give all of her good looks to a girl!

In Hope of Fertility

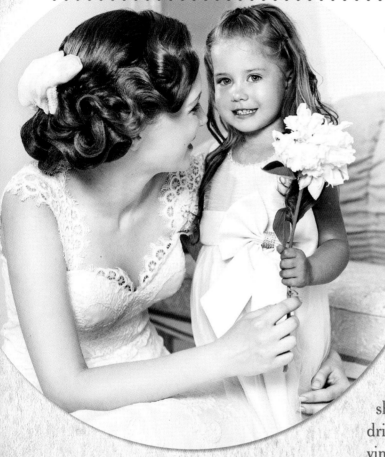

a fertile union. It is good luck to include small children in the wedding party; the presence of infants and children is representative of "sympathetic" magic (like attracting like). Plants and flowers reflect the desire for growth, so the wedding location is sometimes decorated with evergreen boughs as well.

The bride's attire has long been a focus of fertility: There was often a hair from her mother's head taped behind her ear, a wheat pattern sewn on her dress, and bread crumbs placed in her bosom.

A three-part custom says that the couple should eat rice at the wedding for fertility, drink wine for the pleasures of life, and sip vinegar so they will share all of life's bitterness and trouble together. A variation of that custom is for the couple to bring salt, bread, and wine into their new house to insure that they will be fertile and never lack for food or drink. Also to promote fertility, besides being carried by the groom, the bride can carry a baby over the threshold. The couple can also have their mothers make the bed, or they can put a leafy branch or a baby on it. Then they can toast each other and throw the glasses in the fire.

Traditions for fertility fall into two categories. There are customs that are designed to insure fertility and there are practices to deal with the problem of infertility.

Many hopeful symbols of growth and abundance cluster around the marriage ceremony and the early days of a marriage. Throwing rice, corn, or wheat at the wedding, for instance, represents the guests' wishes for

If all these practices failed and the couple was not soon expecting, there were a number of things they could do. The couple could maximize their chances of getting pregnant by making love during a full moon. Also, there were several patent medicines of the past that promised "a baby in every bottle." Or, a sister of the would-be mother could lay her baby on their bed. (It was even luckier if the baby urinated there.) The couple could try putting salt in their bed or garlic under the pillow. Or they could eat the garlic, which is believed to be second only to eggs in promoting fertility. Other recommended foods include oysters (a well-known aphrodisiac), olives, onions, fish, mistletoe juice, cornflower tea, mandrake root, pomegranates, or any many-seeded plant. The wife might try eating three pickled plums a day after sex for one week; the husband could devour a wildcat.

The couple also could turn to magic or religion, such as tying a red ribbon around the finger of a deceased relative to remind him to intercede on their behalf when he appeared before God. One elaborate ritual suggested that the couple learn alternating verses of the story of Genesis in the Bible and repeat them to one other, a verse at a time, on alternate days, just before intercourse.

A very common magical belief was that if a childless couple adopted a child, biological children would follow.

This lore demonstrates the well-known anthropological theory that people resort to magical thinking when events seem beyond their control. It also reveals the deep emotional investment in the idea of children, and how the human imagination works with this universal concern.

Sometimes, of course, it wasn't fertility that was the problem. It was that offspring could grow too numerous. "A poor man will always have many children," goes one saying, which was used to console him for his poverty (or perhaps explain it!). Methods of contraception did not seem to offer much for the overburdened pair, since it is often at odds with biological science: cola or vinegar douches, and coitus while standing, sitting, or with the woman on top. Some women still believe that they are more likely to get pregnant during their period than the rest of the month. This is because they envision their wombs as "open" to let out menstrual flow and "closed" the rest of the month. Of course, the exact opposite, timing-wise, is true.

A pregnant woman can become a source of further fecundity. Perfect strangers may ask to touch her stomach for luck. And, whereas menstruating women, being temporarily "sterile," were supposed to avoid tasks like planting or baking, a pregnant woman might be asked to lend her hand to these types of endeavors where increase was desired.

REMEDIES DURING
PREGNANCY

Raspberry Leaf

Raspberry leaf (*Rubus idaeus, Rubus strigosus*) is probably the most famous natural remedy for use during pregnancy. It has been used in Europe since ancient times to prepare for pregnancy and to nourish the mother during pregnancy. The use of raspberry is still mentioned in the medicine of New York and Michigan and in the Hispanic traditions of the Southwest. It is frequently prescribed as a nourishing beverage for pregnant women by contemporary professional herbalists in North America and Europe.

Raspberry leaf is highly nutritious, especially in the extra minerals and trace elements required during pregnancy. An ounce of the leaf contains 408 milligrams of calcium, 446 milligrams of potassium, 106 milligrams of magnesium, 3.3 milligrams of iron, and 4.0 milligrams of manganese. The concentration of manganese, an essential trace element, is about equal to the recommended dietary allowance for women. Deficiency of manganese has been associated with reproductive disorders in animals. (Neither manganese nor raspberry leaf have been tested in clinical trials of pregnancy outcomes.)

A published review of world literature on herbal safety indicates that raspberry leaf is safe for use during pregnancy. Raspberry leaf can also be taken to settle the stomach in morning sickness. It may relieve nausea through the action of its astringent constituents on the stomach lining.

Directions: Place one ounce of raspberry leaf in one quart of water. Bring to a boil, cover, and simmer for thirty minutes. Strain and drink the quart during the day. Drink as a beverage during the last two trimesters of pregnancy.

Exercise

Exercise is the best tonic for easy delivery, according to the Amish. In William R. McGrath's *Amish Folk Remedies for Plain and Fancy Ailments*, one Amish source said: "Active farm mothers who keep working at home generally have an easier delivery than those who give up all activity and grow fat and flabby."

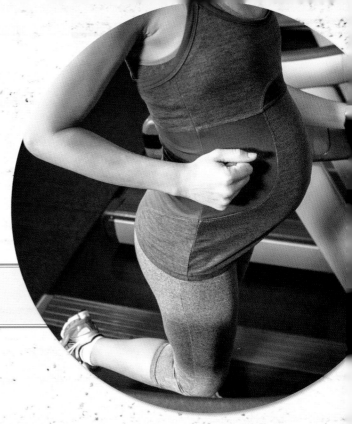

Directions: Engage in moderate daily exercise.

Stinging Nettle Leaf

Leaves of the stinging nettle (*Urtica dioica, Urtica urens*) are a common nutritive herb prescribed by midwives in the New England area and upstate New York. Nettle is one of the most mineral-rich herbs available for common consumption. An ounce of nettle contains more than the minimum daily requirement of calcium, two thirds of the requirement of magnesium, and more than one third of the requirement of potassium.

Directions: Place one ounce of dried nettle leaf in one quart of water and simmer until one third of the liquid is evaporated. Cool and strain. Drink the remaining liquid during the day in three doses every other day in pregnancy.

Ginger

Ginger (*Zingiber officinale*) is used for treating nausea caused by morning sickness in the natural remedies of New England and the Pacific Northwest. One scientific trial demonstrated that ginger is effective against severe morning sickness in doses as low as one gram, or the amount found in two average-sized gelatin capsules. Other clinical trials have shown that ginger may also reduce nausea caused by motion sickness or chemotherapy.

Ginger contains a variety of anti-inflammatory and anesthetic constituents. Huge doses of ginger, such as the ⅓-ounce doses common in traditional Chinese medicine, are contraindicated during pregnancy because of their possible emmenagogue effect (stimulating the flow of menses). The U.S. Food and Drug Administration considers ginger safe for human consumption in doses less than five grams. Take it in the form of tea rather than large amounts of powder, however.

Directions: Place ½ teaspoon of powdered ginger spice in a cup. Fill with boiling water. Cover and let stand for ten minutes. Strain and take in sips, as desired. Don't repeat this more than three times a day during pregnancy. Don't take ginger tea without consulting your doctor if you have gallstones.

Mint

Mints such as peppermint (*Mentha piperita*) and spearmint (*Mentha spicata*) are used throughout North America and Europe for treating nausea. Peppermint was used medicinally by the ancient Egyptians and was valued by the Greeks and Romans. The 16th century British herbalist Nicholas Culpeper claimed that it is one of the best herbal treatments for nausea. German medical texts also list nausea as an indication for the use of mint. Hispanic traditions of the Southwest recommends these herbs specifically for morning sickness. Anesthetic constituents in the mint may reduce nausea by reducing the stomach's gag reflex.

Directions: Place one tablespoon of mint leaves in a one-pint jar and fill with boiling water. Let stand twenty to thirty minutes, shaking the bottle from time to time to mix its contents. Strain and sip as often as desired for nausea.

Prenatal Influences

Modern medicine and folk tradition agree that the health of a pregnant woman directly affects the unborn child. Folk tradition, however, goes much further than the standard clinical advice of a balanced diet and exercise. It asserts that the fetus can be influenced not only by physical health, but by actions, emotions, and events in the life of the mother, and sometimes even the father.

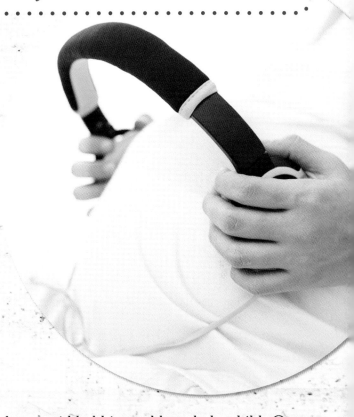

The idea of "marking" a child is the most direct expression of this symbiotic relationship. According to this theory, the baby may be born with some unusual physical or mental trait as a result of something the mother did or didn't do. Food cravings are the most common cause of a child's peculiarity or condition. If a mother craves strawberries and doesn't get them, for instance, the baby might be born with a strawberry birthmark. If she happens to touch herself while thinking of what she wants, the birthmark will be on the same spot on the child. For example, if she touches her shoulder while thinking of chocolate, the child will have a brown mark on his shoulder.

The anthropologist Loudell Snow reports that, in her observation in Michigan prenatal clinics, this belief is so strong that mothers eat food they know isn't good for them (by the clinicians' standards) because they feared that to withhold it would mark the child. One young woman told Dr. Snow that, if a woman craved chicken and didn't get it, the child might have skin like a chicken. Too much of a food, however, can have the same effect—if the mother eats a lot of bananas, the child will have a banana mark, or perhaps a loathing for that fruit.

Another common cause of marking is said to be the result of a shock or fright: A child whose mother is frightened by a cat during pregnancy might look like a cat. (Or, the child will have a lifelong fear of cats.) Any strong emotion or preoccupation has the potential to inflict a mark.

Because of the belief in marking, pregnant women have been advised to use care in what they see and do. Some of the recommendations are strangely specific: "A pregnant woman should never clean fish or her baby will have a fish mouth." More typically, they suggest avoiding potentially upsetting situations such as funerals or horror movies. Instead, to produce a beautiful baby, a pregnant woman should dwell on beautiful things. She should listen to music to produce a musician, study art for an artist, and so on. The father, too, must be careful of his conduct: "If a man calls his pregnant wife a rat, the child will look like a rat."

It should not be surprising that these beliefs are so prevalent. They were part of official medical doctrine in the United States well into the 20th century. These ideas were discarded slightly earlier in Europe, after centuries of acceptance. Hippocrates was said to have saved the day for a white princess who gave birth to a black baby by explaining that there was a picture of a black man in her room.

The idea of parental marking takes on a darker cast in the suggestion that a child may be born with some peculiarity or disability as a punishment for its parents' sins. A Canadian maritime legend tells of a man who shot seagulls or small birds and all his descendants had beady bird-like eyes. The most common transgression is the result of the mother's mocking of someone less fortunate than herself. A woman who made fun of a club-footed man had a child with a clubfoot, for example. A rich woman observing a poor woman and her children remarked, "Doesn't she look like a sow with her litter?" The rich woman's child was born with a pig's hoof for a hand.

Another possible cause of abnormality was the result of a curse put on the child by an enemy of the parents. The idea that a child's abnormality was the result of wrong-doing must have engendered terrible feelings of guilt in parents and a sad legacy for the child. Some children were even hidden from society out of a sense of shame.

Some ideas about prenatal influences were of a purely physical nature. Reaching above the head—to hang clothes or get something from a cupboard, for instance—was feared to cause the umbilical cord to wrap around the baby's neck. Repetitive motions, like working a treadle sewing machine, might be avoided for the same reason.

Concern for the unborn infant is at the heart of all prenatal folk belief, however farfetched it may seem. Pregnant women can hardly be blamed when they wonder about some of these older ideas.

SKIN

More remedies appear for treating skin problems than for any other type of condition.

The reason why treatments for skin conditions are so plentiful is because skin ailments, although usually minor as far as health risk is concerned, are so common. But skin conditions are also visible and uncomfortable and demand our attention.

Over time, useless natural remedies for the skin were smoothly weeded out—many were topical remedies, so it was usually obvious whether they worked or not. People kept the skin remedies that worked effectively and incorporated them into tradition.

Elsewhere in this book we cover acne, athlete's foot, bites and stings, boils and carbuncles, burns and sunburn, eczema, itching and rashes, and poison ivy and poison oak. In this section, we'll discuss remedies for heat rash, chapped skin, and impetigo as well as remedies designed for better overall health of the skin.

Of the conditions here, impetigo is the most serious. Impetigo is a skin condition that may be caused by *Staphylococcus* or *Streptococcus* bacteria. And, because of decades of antibiotic overuse, antibiotic-resistant strains of these bacteria are now common. It is possible, although rare, that an antibiotic-resistant strain of the bacteria might cause a systemic infection. Any infection of the skin that develops red streaks around it requires immediate medical attention.

From the Inside Out

Some common folk remedies fall into the traditional category of "blood purifiers." Traditional "blood tonic" herbs mentioned in the folk literature for skin conditions are red clover, burdock, boneset, sarsaparilla, and wild cherry bark. The idea of blood purifiers has a solid physiological basis because the skin receives all of its nutrients from the blood. Thus, these herbs are used to treat the skin "from the inside out." In the same way, toxins, allergens, or irritants in the blood can also cause symptoms of skin infection.

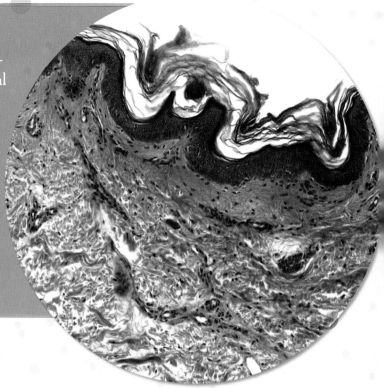

Scarred for Life?

Reduction or elimination of scars is a common human desire, and remedies to reduce scarring appear in several North American traditions. Scars result from wound healing or from inflammation. This natural process leaves the injured tissue stronger than it was before the injury. Most agents that suppress scar formation, herbal or not, also tend to suppress healing. Treatments must be applied as soon as the wound is closed. Coconut oil, cocoa butter, castor oil, and vitamin E oil are all used as natural remedies.

Salves & Ointments

Homemade salves and ointments are commonly used throughout the world. To make one, a medicinal plant is cooked or mixed in lard, butter, beeswax, or other oily substance that remains solid at room temperature. The oily portion of the salve helps to soften and penetrate the tissues and also serves to hold the medicinal portion in place. To make a simple salve, chop, powder, crush, or grind the medicinal material as small as possible and place in the bottom of a skillet or a crock pot. Place enough lard, butter, or beeswax in the pan or pot; it should cover the plant material when melted. Leave on very lowest heat for a while—at least ten to twenty minutes for a leafy substance, forty to sixty minutes for roots. Remove from heat. Let the ointment cool to a solid state. Store lard or butter ointments in the refrigerator. Plantain, grindelia, goldenseal, rosemary, and osha are all easy to make into salves. Combinations of the herbs may make more effective salves than single herb preparations.

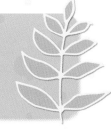

Remedies for the Skin

Red Clover

Red clover (*Trifolium pratense*) is a commonly used remedy for treating skin conditions (such as acne, eczema, boils, and rashes). It can be applied externally, which is recorded in the traditions of Indiana, or it can be taken as a tea, which is the practice in the southern Appalachian region.

Red clover tea is also one of the most often prescribed remedies for skin conditions in professional medical herbalism in North America. Red clover was used both internally and externally for skin conditions by the Eclectic physicians at the turn of the century. Harvey Felter, M.D., an Eclectic professor of medicine, said in his *King's American Dispensatory* that red clover, when applied externally, soothes inflamed skin, disinfects it, and promotes the growth of healthy tissue.

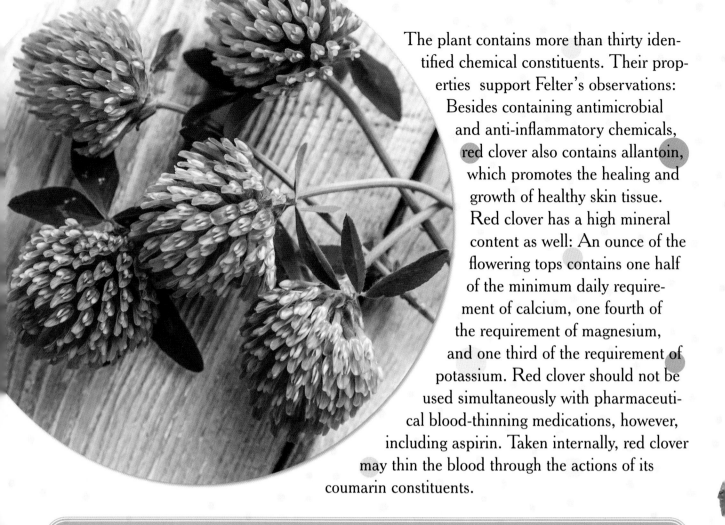

The plant contains more than thirty iden-tified chemical constituents. Their prop-erties support Felter's observations: Besides containing antimicrobial and anti-inflammatory chemicals, red clover also contains allantoin, which promotes the healing and growth of healthy skin tissue. Red clover has a high mineral content as well: An ounce of the flowering tops contains one half of the minimum daily require-ment of calcium, one fourth of the requirement of magnesium, and one third of the requirement of potassium. Red clover should not be used simultaneously with pharmaceuti-cal blood-thinning medications, however, including aspirin. Taken internally, red clover may thin the blood through the actions of its coumarin constituents.

Directions: To treat the skin from the inside out, add one ounce of red clover tops to one quart of water. Simmer on the lowest possible heat until one third of the water is gone. Cool and strain. Drink the liquid in three doses during the day.

For external use, try this remedy from Indiana: Simmer whole flowering red clover plants until tender. Use just enough water to cover. Strain, press the plants into a thick mass, and sprinkle with white flour. (The flour helps add consistency to the poultice.) Place the floured poultice directly on the irritated skin. Leave on for about half an hour. You can use the red clover poultice several times a day. (The poultice can last a few days if it's kept in the refrigerator between applications.) The poultice is designed to help reduce inflammation and promote healing.

Jojoba Oil

The Papago Indian tribe of the Southwest has used jojoba nut (*Simmondsia chinensis*) preparations to treat skin conditions such as boils and rashes. The nuts are traditionally dried and then pulverized and applied to the skin. Jojoba oil is now commercially extracted, and it is a popular addition to skin creams, oils, and ointments available in health food stores. The oil is also used today in the traditional medicine of the Southwest for chapped skin.

Directions: Apply commercial jojoba oil as desired to dry, chapped skin.

Plantain Leaves

Plantain leaves (*Plantago major*) are a common weed found on lawns throughout the United States. It was naturalized in North America after the arrival of the Europeans. American Indians called it "White Man's Footprint" because it seemed to follow the European colonists wherever they went. The Delaware, Mohegan, Ojibwa, Cherokee, and other American Indian tribes used plantain for treating minor wounds and insect bites.

Plantain has been used in cultures around the world to treat wounds and skin conditions. Plantain contains a pharmacy of constituents that are beneficial to the skin, including at least fifteen anti-inflammatory constituents and six analgesic chemicals. Like red clover, it contains the constituent allantoin, which promotes cell proliferation and tissue healing.

Directions: Crush a small handful of fresh plantain leaves and apply the juice locally to dry, chapped skin.

Vinegar

Vinegar is also a remedy for chapped hands, according to folklorist Clarence Meyer's *American Folk Medicine*. The Amish use vinegar and water to treat heat rash in babies. No scientific reason for such a treatment is apparent.

Directions: After washing and drying the hands thoroughly, apply vinegar, put on a pair of gloves, and go to bed.

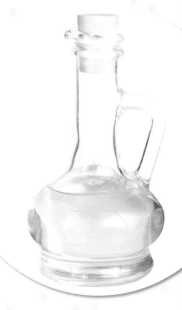

Urine

Using your own urine as a treatment for chapped hands is part of the folklore of New England. Urine is also used for chapping in the folklore of Hispanics in the Southwest and among blacks in Louisiana. Urine therapy for cleansing wounds and treating skin infections appeared in the ancient medical systems of Mexico, Egypt, Persia, India, and China. It was used in 17th and 18th century Europe as well. Urine contains the substance urea, a disinfectant and skin moistener used in modern pharmaceutical preparations to cleanse wounds and in cosmetic products. (It is animal urine that is used in these preparations, of course.)

Directions: Apply fresh warm urine to chapped hands and skin and allow skin to air dry.

Oatmeal

Oatmeal is a treatment for chapped hands in folklorist Clarence Meyer's collection of remedies called *American Folk Medicine*. In the method described below, oatmeal is used to both moisten and dry the skin.

Directions: Use wet oatmeal instead of soap to wash chapped hands. Then, after drying hands with a towel, rub the hands with dry oatmeal.

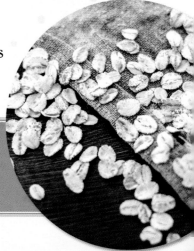

Clay

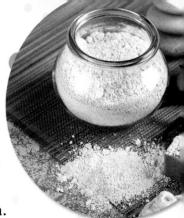

Clay application is a common natural remedy for treating various skin conditions throughout the world. It was common among the North American Indians even before the arrival of the European colonists. Today, the therapeutic use of clay makes up an important part of modern Seventh Day Adventist traditions. Clay is drawing and cooling. It is most effective on moist and inflamed conditions rather than on dry, chapped skin.

Directions: Purchase bentonite clay or cosmetic grade clay at a health food store or drugstore. Mix the clay with water to make a paste and apply to the skin. Allow to dry, then gently flake off after a few hours. Wipe the clay off over a bowl. Discard the waste in your garden or on your lawn, because clay can stop up your pipes. Apply clay every few hours.

Goldenseal

Goldenseal (*Hydrastis canadensis*) was used as an American Indian remedy for skin infections, such as impetigo, even before the European colonists arrived. Its use as a topical disinfectant and internal bitter tonic spread rapidly to the English colonists in the eastern parts of the country. It has been used in one school of American medicine or another ever since. Goldenseal contains the antimicrobial substance berberine, which kills both *Streptococcus* and *Staphylococcus* bacteria, the two most common infecting agents in impetigo. Other berberine-containing plants include Oregon grape root (*Mahonia aquifolium, Berberis aquifolium*) and barberry (*Berberis vulgaris*).

Directions: Place ½ ounce of goldenseal root bark or powder in one pint of water. Bring to a boil, then simmer for twenty minutes. Allow the water to cool to room temperature. Stir and, without straining, apply to the affected area with a clean cloth. Cover with a clean bandage or gauze pad. Reapply the application every two hours as desired.

Skin

Gumweed

Gumweed (*Grindelia* spp.) grows throughout the American Southwest and northwestern Mexico. It has been used as a skin remedy in those regions first by the American Indians and later by others who settled there.

Gumweed entered into the medical practice of the Eclectic physicians during the late 19th and early 20th centuries. In *The Eclectic Materia Medica, Pharmacology, and Therapeutics*, Harvey Felter, M.D., an Eclectic professor of medicine, states that gumweed was especially well-suited to treat those skin conditions characterized by "feeble circulation and a tendency to ulceration."

Gumweed was an official medicine in the United States Pharmacopoeia from 1882 until 1926. It remains an official medicine in Germany; it is used there as an expectorant for coughs. Little research has been performed into the constituents of gumweed. The resin contains anti-inflammatory constituents, so it may be useful in treating infectious or inflammatory skin conditions.

Directions: Apply the sticky sap from the leaves or flowers of gumweed to the affected areas. Reapply every few hours. Alternately, you can purchase some tincture of gumweed and use it as a wash. Reapply the tincture every few hours.

Garlic Paste

In Romani traditions garlic is used as a treatment for all types of skin infections, including impetigo, cuts, and wounds. When garlic is cut or crushed, it releases a substance called allicin, one of the most potent broad-spectrum antimicrobial chemicals known. This same substance, which is part of the plant's defense system against bacteria, virus, molds, and yeast, is responsible for the burning effect of fresh cut garlic.

Directions: Pulverize three cloves of garlic in a blender or with a mortar and pestle. Add vinegar a drop at a time to make a thin paste that can be applied to the infected area. Apply twice a day, leaving in place for ten to fifteen minutes each time. This preparation can cause skin burns, including severe blistering, so don't exceed the recommended time limit. Afterward, wash the area thoroughly and cover the area with a clean dressing.

Rosemary

Rosemary leaf (*Rosmarinus officinalis*) is a remedy from the Southwest for treating windburn and cracked and chapped skin. It is also used in that region (and other areas as well) as a wash for infectious skin conditions. The plant's leaf contains four anti-inflammatory substances—carnosol, oleanolic acid, rosmarinic acid, and ursolic acid. Rosemary also contains more than ten antiseptic constituents.

Directions: Crush some rosemary leaves and warm in a pan on low heat. Add some lard to make a salve. Simmer over low heat until the lard takes on the color and aroma of the rosemary.

Let cool. Apply to the affected areas as desired.

Alternately, place one ounce of crushed rosemary leaf in a one-pint jar and fill with boiling water. Cover tightly and let stand until the water reaches room temperature. Apply as a wash to the affected area, using a clean cloth, as often as desired.

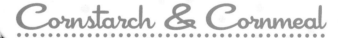

Cornstarch & Cornmeal

Cornstarch and cornmeal are common agents used to treat moist skin conditions such as heat rash, according to folklorist Clarence Meyer's *American Folk Medicine*. Cornstarch and cornmeal are also used to treat chapped skin and prickly heat. Cornstarch "dusting powder" appears in the contemporary folklore of Indiana.

Directions: Wash the affected area, wipe it dry, and dust with cornstarch.

Skin

Vitamin E Oil

Vitamin E oil rubbed into scar tissue will help to reduce a scar, according to the traditions of the Amish. The Amish also use cocoa butter and castor oil for the same purpose. All three oils contain vitamin E, but the vitamin E oil contains higher amounts. Vitamin E has been shown to reduce scarring in a variety of scientific experiments. Treatment with vitamin E for skin grafts after severe burns did not work in one trial, however, so there may be a limit as to what can be accomplished with this simple remedy.

Directions: As soon as possible after a wound is closed, rub vitamin E oil (or one of the other oils above) into the tissues for five to ten minutes twice a day. The rubbing, which increases circulation and can break up deep scars, is an important part of the application process. Continue rubbing in the oil on a daily basis for months if necessary, or at least until improvement appears.

Potato Poultice

According to medical traditions of the Romani, a potato poultice will improve puffy skin, especially those "bags" under the eyes. This same method is taught in contemporary naturopathic medical schools to reduce inflammation of the skin.

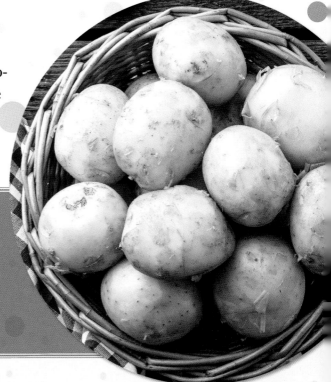

Directions: Thoroughly clean two or three potatoes. Grate (including the potato skins) and press them with your hands into a paste. Apply to the affected areas of the skin. Leave in place while relaxing for fifteen minutes. Remove the poultice and clean and dry the area.

Milk

Milk is applied to the skin to relieve the irritation and discomfort of a variety of skin ailments in the traditions of the Hispanic Southwest. The remedy is also popular in the medicine of New England. In the southern Appalachians, it is buttermilk that's preferred. These remedies traditionally used whole milk right from the cow, which, these days, is not usually available for sale. If you're going to try this remedy, use whole milk, not low fat milk. The short- and medium-chain fatty acids in the butterfat of whole milk may have a mild antimicrobial effect on the skin. Any beneficial effect of this remedy is more likely due to the soothing quality of the milk rather than any actual pharmaceutical activity.

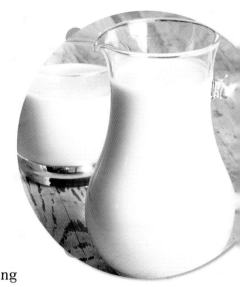

Directions: Wash the affected area with milk or buttermilk as desired.

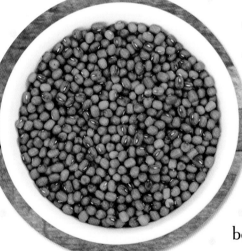

Mung Bean Paste

A treatment for heat rash or prickly heat from Chinese folklore is mung bean "soap," which is made from a mixture of cooked mung beans and sugar. The most important component of the formula may be the sugar, however, because by nature it is drying and cooling. Sugar has been used in various cultures to cleanse wounds. The astringent and drying properties of the beans may also have a beneficial effect on the rash.

Directions: Cook mung beans until they can be mashed into the consistency of a paste. Add enough sugar so that the beans are sweet to the taste. Apply to the affected area, rubbing as if the paste were soap. Leave the paste in place for ten to fifteen minutes. Then remove, dry the area well, and dust with talcum powder or another drying agent.

Skin

Watermelon Rind

To treat rash in babies, the Amish suggest rubbing the affected area with watermelon rind.

Directions: Rub the affected area with the inside of a watermelon rind. Be sure to dry the area thoroughly and apply a talcum powder or some other drying agent.

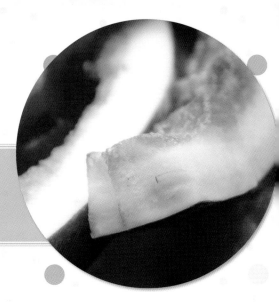

Osha

Osha (*Ligusticum porteri*), which is native to the Rocky Mountains, was a panacea to the American Indians in the area. The plant remains one of the most important natural remedies of the residents of the Rio Grande Valley. Osha is used for colds, flu, bronchitis, and also as a skin wash for superficial infections.

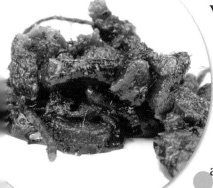

Very little scientific research has been performed into either the constituents or the pharmaceutical properties of the plant, but a close Chinese relative of the plant (*Ligusticum wallichi*) has been studied extensively. The main constituent of its aromatic oil is alpha-pinene, which has antimicrobial and disinfectant properties. Constituents called ligustilides, which are common to both the North American and Chinese species, have broad spectrum antibiotic effects as well as antiviral and antifungal properties.

Directions: Using a coffee grinder, grind a piece of osha root into a powder. Spread the powder in a small skillet. Add enough lard or butter to cover the powder when melted. Put on low heat until the lard or butter is melted. Stir well and let stand at room temperature until the salve becomes solid. To treat a skin infection, apply the salve to the skin every two to three hours.

Alternately, mix the osha with enough honey to make a paste. Apply to a piece of gauze and use a bandage to hold in place over the affected area. Osha may irritate the skin. If this occurs, reduce the frequency of the treatments or try another remedy.

Sweating It Out

Many natural remedies aim to provoke heavy perspiration, although it is seldom known why this is done. The implicit principle seems to be that the body leaches dangerous substances along with the sweat, which may explain why at one time sweat was thought to be poisonous. "Cleaning the blood" was a common phrase used with these cures (replaced today by "ridding the body of toxins"). A hot drink was usually the first step to getting things flowing: teas of sassafras root, bitter orange, and boneset (alias "sweatweed") were just a few of the suggested infusions. Many of the medicinal recipes included alcohol; one cure bypasses drinking the beverage altogether and suggests rubbing the person with whisky until he sweats. In Hawaii, persons with fever would lie under a blanket of ti leaves until they sweated to "break the fever."

Sweating it out—whatever "it" is—may or may not be a good idea in the case of fever, however. Certain organisms cannot survive in an abnormally high body temperature, and some doctors now suggest that reducing a fever may hinder the body's efforts to heal itself. By this logic, to elevate a fever even more, as the cures suggest, could conceivably speed the process along. A high fever can be dangerous, however, and pushing one even higher seems extreme.

The idea of sweating as a healthful and cleansing process is found in many cultures. Some even build special structures for sweat-baths: The Russian have the *bania*; the Greeks have the *laconica*; and many American-Indian groups have the *maquiq*.

Sweat-bathing practices often have social and spiritual significance in addition to their hygienic function. Finnish immigrants used the sauna as a place to get clean and to meet friends each week. The sauna is considered essential to health: "If sauna, brandy, nor tar helps, the disease is of death," according to an American-Finnish proverb.

Healing Diaphoretics

Many traditional natural remedies are called diaphoretics—plants or foods that make you sweat. Constituents in these plants increase the blood circulation to the skin, which, when taken internally, can be helpful in healing various skin conditions. Some diaphoretics are recommended for common skin ailments in the folklore of the southern Appalachian mountains. For example, burdock, boneset, elder flowers, and yarrow have all been used in folklore there to treat skin conditions "from the inside out" by increasing circulation to the skin.

Skin

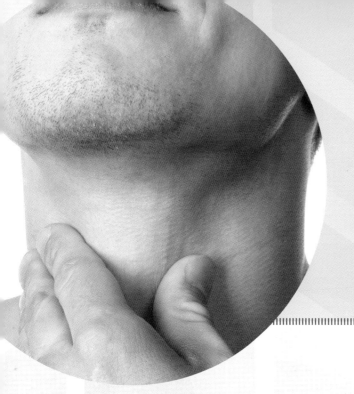

SORE THROAT

A sore throat can be a minor, but annoying, ailment—or it can be a symptom of a serious illness.

A sore throat is a painful irritation in the throat. A sore throat can range from mild scratchiness to severe pain and difficulty in swallowing.

A sore throat is most frequently seen as a symptom of a virus. When an individual suffers from a common cold, the nasal passages are congested and the person is forced to breathe through the mouth, leaving the throat dry and irritated. Coughing may also irritate the throat, as will the secretions that drain into the throat from the back of the nose during a cold.

A severe sore throat may be caused by a bacterial (usually *Streptococcus* bacteria, or strep) infection of the throat, middle

ear, or sinuses. It is difficult to determine from the symptoms whether a sore throat is due to a virus or to strep (although a doctor can tell the difference using laboratory tests). Both infections may be accompanied by fever, headache, and fatigue, and both infections normally get better on their own. The fever subsides within a few days, the sore throat improves, and all signs of infection are usually gone within two weeks.

The complications of a strep throat begin between one and six weeks after the first appearance of the sore throat, usually after about two weeks. For this reason, any sore throat that lasts more than a week requires a visit to the doctor. A number of individuals who carry *Streptococcus* bacteria are without any symptoms at all. In fact, twenty percent of children are carriers, and most are asymptomatic. Concern for complications comes only with active inflammation, although the symptoms may seem minor.

Strep throat can have serious complications, however. A prolonged strep infection can result in damage to the heart (called rheumatic fever) or to the kidneys. These complications are rare, however—less than one percent of strep throats result in these illnesses. But the complications are common enough to warrant antibiotic prescriptions for strep infections, which is the standard treatment in modern medicine. Antibiotics for strep also reduce secondary infections, such as ear infection or pneumonia, that might accompany the sore throat. (Antibiotics are of no value in sore throats caused by these viruses.)

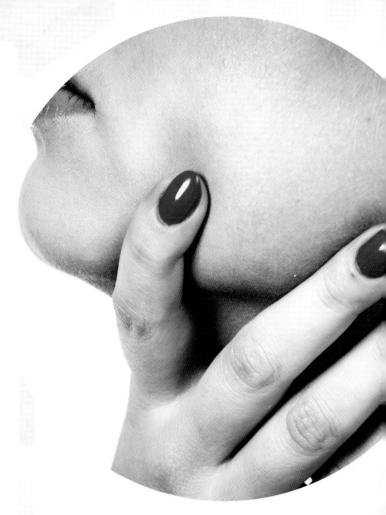

Natural remedy treatments for sore throats fall into five categories. First, there are remedies that act as astringents, which reduce swelling of the mucous membrane tissues and thereby reduce pain. Second, there are demulcents such as slippery elm. These herbs or foods have a slimy constituency that is soothing to inflamed tissues. The third category contains plants used to treat sore throat like goldenseal or garlic that are antibacterial and antiviral. In the fourth category are the remedies such as mint and echinacea that contain

local anesthetics that help numb a sore throat. Finally, many of the herbs used in natural remedies for sore throat contain anti-inflammatory constituents that may reduce pain and swelling. Most of the remedies combine more than one of these actions. For example, sage leaf is both astringent and antiseptic. Mint is both antiseptic and anesthetic. Willow bark is both astringent and anti-inflammatory. Most remedies call for gargling the substance, and most can be swallowed after gargling for further benefits.

Remedies for
SORE THROAT

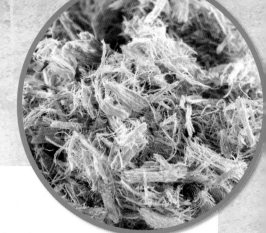

Slippery Elm

Slippery elm bark (*Ulmus* spp., *Ulmus fulva*) was used to treat
sore throats by members of at least six American Indian tribes, including
the Iroquois and the Cherokee, even before the arrival of the European colonists. Slippery elm has been a natural treatment for sore throat in the United States at least since
the early 1800s when its use was popularized by the Thomsonian herbalists. Slippery
elm was an official remedy in the United States Pharmacopoeia from 1820 until 1930.
Slippery elm throat lozenges have been sold throughout the United States since the late
1800s. They are available today in many health food stores and pharmacies. Slippery
elm powder, when moistened, has a slimy quality that is soothing to inflamed mucous
membranes. Professional medical herbalists in the United States, Australia, and Europe
use slippery elm to soothe inflammations of the mouth, throat, and intestines. Its use continues today in the medicine of New England, North Carolina, and Indiana.

Directions: Place one tablespoon of powdered slippery elm bark in a cup. Fill with
boiling water. Let steep for ten minutes. Stir, without straining, and first gargle, then
swallow ½-cup doses to soothe a sore throat. Do this as often as desired.

Alternately, make honey lozenges of slippery elm by mixing the slippery elm powder with
hot honey. Spread the paste on a marble slab or other nonstick surface coated with sugar
or cornstarch. With a rolling pin, roll the mixture flat to about the thickness of a pancake.
Sprinkle with sugar and cornstarch. With a knife, cut into small, separate squares. Or
pinch off pieces and roll into ¼-inch balls. Flatten the balls into round lozenges. Allow
lozenges to air-dry in a well-ventilated area for twelve hours. Then store them in the
refrigerator. Suck on lozenges to help heal sore throats.

Also, the most basic method, mentioned in several natural remedy traditions, is to chew on
the bark and swallow the juice or suck on the plain bark powder.

Red Root

Red root (*Ceanothus americanus, Ceanothus* spp.) was used for a wide variety of ailments, including colds and coughs, by American Indians living in the regions where it grows. Eclectic and Physiomedicalist physicians adopted the use of red root in the mid-19th century. A tea of the leaves was used during the Civil War as a treatment for malaria. Today, red root is used to treat sore throats in the medicine of Appalachia and by Hispanics in the Southwest.

Red root is astringent like black tea and was even used as a substitute for tea during the Civil War when black tea was unavailable. Some *Ceanothus* species contain a small amount of caffeine. Red root also contains anti-inflammatory and antimicrobial constituents that may help soothe and disinfect a sore throat. Its constituents ceanothic acid and ceanothetric acid have specifically shown to inhibit the growth of *Streptococcus* bacteria in laboratory experiments. (A tincture must be used, rather than a tea, to take advantage of the anti-streptococcal activity, however.) Red root has not been tested in clinical trials. The tea is a better source of the astringent constituents than the tincture and is the form used by physicians during the last century.

Directions: Simmer one ounce of red root in one pint of water on low heat for twenty minutes. Let cool to room temperature. Gargle doses of one tablespoon and swallow, four times a day. Alternately, you can purchase a tincture of red root at a health food store or herb shop. Hold a teaspoon dose of the tincture in the mouth and swish it around. Then gargle and swallow. Do this four times a day for as long as necessary.

Goldenseal

Goldenseal (*Hydrastis canadensis*) was a sore throat remedy among eastern American Indian tribes. The colonists quickly adopted the plant as a household medicine and by the 1830s physicians were using it to treat sore throats. Goldenseal was an official medicine in the United States Pharmacopoeia from 1840 until 1920. It is still used today to treat sore throats in the medicine of North Carolina.

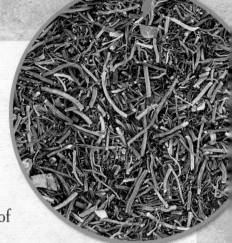

The plant's constituent berberine is a strong antibiotic—about as potent as pharmaceutical drugs of the sulfa group. Berberine must come in direct contact with microorganisms in order to kill them, and it does not enter the bloodstream the way most pharmaceutical antibiotics do. Oregon grape root (*Mahonia aquifolium, Berberis aquifolium*) and barberry (*Berberis vulgaris*) also contain berberine. (Both plants were used for treating sore throats by American Indians in the regions where they grow.) Of the three plants, goldenseal is probably best for treating sore throats because, unlike the other two plants, it contains powerful astringents. However, goldenseal is now an endangered species and is very expensive. Oregon grape root and barberry root, on the other hand, are inexpensive and plentiful.

Directions: Place one ounce of one of the above roots in a pint of water. Bring to a boil and simmer on the lowest heat for twenty minutes. Let cool to room temperature. Gargle and swallow doses of one to two tablespoons three to four times a day.

Oak Bark

Oak bark (*Quercus* spp.) has been used to treat sore throats since antiquity in European medicine. In this country, oak bark was used for the same purpose by members of the Delaware, Cherokee, Houma, Alabama, and Iroquois Indian tribes. Later, from 1820 until 1930, oak bark was an official medicine in the United States Pharmacopoeia.

Oak bark contains a high level of tannins—the same substances found in black tea. Oak bark is mentioned today in the medicine of North Carolina. It is also used by professional medical herbalists in North America and Europe.

Directions: Boil three tablespoons of oak bark in one pint of water for twenty minutes. Let cool and strain. Gargle with one or two tablespoons of the tea three to four times a day for as long as necessary.

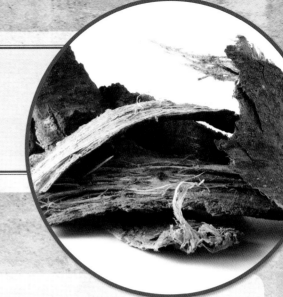

Horehound

A natural remedy for sore throats from contemporary Indiana is horehound (*Marrubium vulgare*). Horehound has been used in European medicine since the time of the ancient Greeks. It was later used for treating sore throats in this country by the Mahuna and Navaho Indian tribes. Horehound became an official cough remedy in the United States Pharmacopoeia between 1840 and 1910. It remains an approved medicine for coughs by the German government today.

The herb is most famous as a cough medicine. Horehound cough drops are available in some health food stores and pharmacies. Besides its expectorant properties, horehound also contains astringent tannins (like those in tea) and anti-inflammatory and antimicrobial aromatic oils.

Directions: Place one tablespoon of dried horehound in a cup and fill with boiling water. Cover and let steep for fifteen minutes. Strain and sweeten with honey. Gargle ½-cup doses as desired.

Sore Throat

Licorice

A natural remedy from China for sore throats is licorice tea. Licorice is used as a medicine in every major traditional medical system in the world. Extracts of licorice were originally used to make licorice candy, but the spice anise is used for that purpose today. Licorice was an official medicine in the United States Pharmacopoeia from 1820 until 1975; it was listed as a flavoring agent and a demulcent and expectorant for cough syrups.

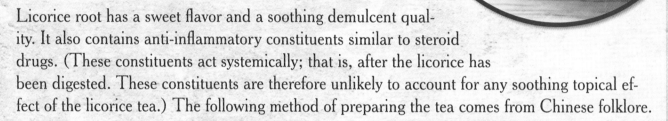

Licorice root has a sweet flavor and a soothing demulcent quality. It also contains anti-inflammatory constituents similar to steroid drugs. (These constituents act systemically; that is, after the licorice has been digested. These constituents are therefore unlikely to account for any soothing topical effect of the licorice tea.) The following method of preparing the tea comes from Chinese folklore.

> **Directions:** Place ½ ounce of licorice root in one quart of water. Boil on low heat in an uncovered pot until half the water has evaporated. Drink the remaining pint in two doses during the course of a day. Repeat for up to three days. Don't take licorice if you are taking steroid drugs.

Rose Bush

A sore throat remedy in the Hispanic tradition of the Southwest is a tea of rose petals (*Rosa* spp.). Rose petals have also been used by American Indians of the Costanoan, Skagut, and Snohomish tribes to treat throat problems. In addition, rose petals are among the top ten of the most often prescribed herbs in contemporary Arabic medicine.

The petals have a strong astringent action and can tone up swollen and inflamed mucous membranes, which is their chief medicinal use in Arabic medicine. The rose oil that gives the flowers their scent also contains antimicrobial and anti-inflammatory substances. The petals are considered to be "cooling" in Arabic medicine, indicating that clinical anti-inflammatory effects have been observed in their medical traditions.

Directions: Pour one pint of boiling water over a handful of rose petals in a one-pint jar. Cover well to retain the aromatic oils, and let stand until the water reaches room temperature. Gargle ½-cup doses as desired for sore throat. Avoid commercial roses and roses that have been sprayed with strong pesticides.

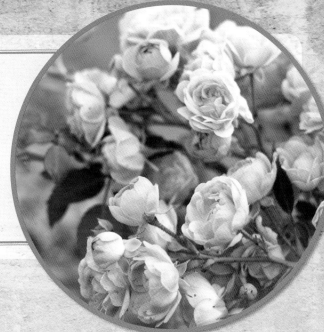

Sage Leaf

Another sore throat remedy from Indiana is sage tea (*Salvia officinalis*), which is made from the common kitchen spice. Sage is a strong astringent, and it also contains anti-inflammatory and antimicrobial aromatic oils. Cultivated garden sage has been used as a medicine in the Mediterranean region since the time of the ancient Egyptians. It is a common remedy for sore throat in the professional medical herbalism of Europe and North America. It is an approved medicine for sore throats in Germany.

Directions: Place one tablespoon of sage leaf in a cup and fill with boiling water. Cover and let stand until it reaches room temperature. Gargle ¼-cup doses three to four times a day for sore throats for as long as necessary. The concentrated essential oil of sage, or the alcohol tincture, should not be taken during pregnancy.

Sore Throat

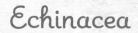

Echinacea

Echinacea (*Echinacea angustifolia*) was used by the Plains Indians for a wide variety of infectious diseases. The Cheyenne, Comanche, and Kiowa all used the herb to treat sore throats. Constituents in the angustifolia species can offer some relief from sore throat pain by producing a tingling and numbness in the mouth and throat that can last for more than half an hour. (These local anesthetic effects are not present in *Echinacea purpurea*, the species used in most of the commercial echinacea products, however. The root or powder of the *Echinacea angustifolia* species is sometimes available, however.) In addition, echinacea is an immune stimulant. It may help the body fight the infection that is causing the sore throat.

Directions: Obtain whole or chopped *Echinacea angustifolia* root at a health food store or herb shop. Grind a small amount in a coffee grinder. Stir ½ teaspoon of the powder into two ounces of warm water. Gargle the water, powder and all, for as long as you can, allowing the powder to coat your throat and mouth.

Mint

Both the Chinese and the Paiute Indians used mint teas (*Mentha* spp.) when treating sore throats. Mint contains a number of anti-inflammatory, antimicrobial, and local anesthetic constituents. The eight anesthetic constituents it contains may provide immediate (but temporary) relief from the pain of sore throat.

Directions: Place one ounce of peppermint leaves in a one-pint jar and fill with boiling water. Cover tightly and let the tea cool, shaking the bottle from time to time to mix the contents. Gargle ½-cup doses of the tea as desired.

Herbal Steam

An entry in folklorist Clarence Meyer's collection of remedies, called *American Folk Medicine*, suggests inhaling steam from an herbal tea to treat severely painful sore throats. The herbs included are sage (*Salvia officinalis*), boneset (*Eupatorium perfoliatum*), catnip (*Nepeta cataria*), hop (*Humulus lupulus*), and horehound (*Marrubium vulgare*). The mixture contains anti-inflammatory and antiviral aromatic oils that presumably can rise with the steam and affect the throat. The steam itself may be antiviral. Most of the viruses that infect the mucous membranes cannot survive at temperatures equal to those in the body's core—about 98.6 degrees Fahrenheit. Thus, the viruses remain at the cooler membranes, near the surface of the body (in the mucous membranes of the respiratory tract). Inhaling hot steam may kill the viruses on contact.

Directions: Place a handful each of sage, boneset, catnip, hop, and horehound in a large bowl. Pour one quart of boiling water over the herbs and inhale the steam that rises, being careful not to burn yourself. If you don't have one or two of the herbs in the formula, use the ones mentioned that you do have.

Willow

Willow bark (*Salix* spp.) is used as an astringent gargle for sore throats in the Hispanic medicine of the Southwest. The same method has been used by the Cherokee and Iroquois Indians and also by the Alaskan Eskimos. Willow bark is astringent. It also contains aspirin-like compounds that may help reduce a fever.

Directions: Simmer three tablespoons of willow bark in one pint of water for twenty to thirty minutes. Gargle with ½-cup doses as desired throughout the day as often as necessary.

Osha

Osha (*Ligusticum porteri*), a Rocky Mountain plant, was used for a variety of ailments by American Indians living in that region. Osha remains one of the most important natural remedies of American Indians and Hispanic residents of the upper Rio Grande Valley in New Mexico and Colorado. A traditional herbalist of the area, Michael Moore, recommends the tea below for sore throat. Osha contains disinfectant aromatic oils and local anesthetic aromatic oils. One of its constituents has antibacterial and antiviral properties.

Directions: Grind an osha root in a coffee grinder. Place one teaspoon of the powder in a cup and fill with boiling water. Cover tightly and allow to stand until the water reaches room temperature. Gargle ¼- to ½-cup doses as desired.

Alternately, mix the powdered osha with enough hot honey to make a paste. Roll the paste into balls as big around as dimes. Store the balls in the refrigerator, where they will cool to a more solid consistency. Suck on the lozenges for sore throat. You can do this as often as desired.

Onion Syrup

Here's a recipe from New England for onion syrup that is remarkably similar to a recipe from North Carolina. The New England recipe calls for sliced raw onions to be placed in a bowl and covered with sugar. Allow the onion to stand until a syrup forms. Adding water is not necessary because the sugar draws the onion juice out of the onions. (It may take a day or two for the syrup to form, however.) The method used in North Carolina is similar, but the onion-and-sugar mixture is placed in a baking pan and baked in the oven until the syrup forms. (Baking presumably speeds up the process.) The onions contain antimicrobial substances, which attack the organisms that are causing the infection. These substances are the same ones that give an onion its odor, and they are also responsible for the burning sensation your eyes feel after you slice an onion.

Directions: Fill a bowl or baking pan with raw onions. Pour enough sugar over them to cover. Then, either let them stand or bake them on medium heat, depending on how fast you need the syrup. Take the syrup in single tablespoon doses as often as desired.

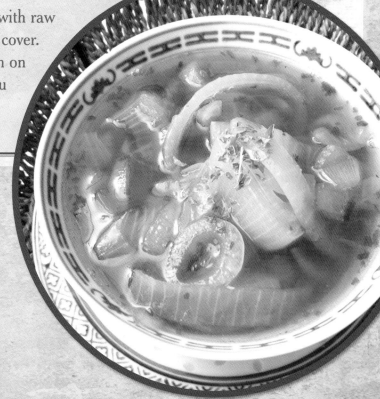

Myrrh Gum

Myrrh gum (*Commiphora myrrha*) has been used as a disinfectant in the Mediterranean region since the time of the ancient Egyptians. Its use spread to India, China, and Europe along Arab trade routes. Its use as a disinfectant was popularized throughout the eastern United States by the Thomsonian herbalists of the early 1800s. Myrrh gum is a powerful antiseptic and it is also astringent—both properties are beneficial to a throat infection.

Directions: Fill a bowl or baking pan with raw onions. Pour enough sugar over them to cover. Then, either let them stand or bake them on medium heat, depending on how fast you need the syrup. Take the syrup in single tablespoon doses as often as desired.

255

Cold Compress

A hydrotherapy treatment from North Carolina traditions calls for applying a cold wet compress to the throat and covering it with a dry one. The method is also used in the Seventh Day Adventist healing tradition. The treatment has its roots in the nature cure and hydrotherapy traditions of Germany, brought to North America by German immigrants near the turn of the 20th century.

Directions: Soak a cotton cloth in cold water. Wring it out and wrap it around the front of the neck below the ears. Be careful to avoid chilling the back of the neck. Wrap a warm wool scarf around the cold cloth and lie down. The cold cloth will supposedly attract circulation to the area, which in turn, promotes healing of the throat. The body will usually heat the cold cloth in twenty to forty minutes. Repeat the treatment two to four times each day.

Garlic

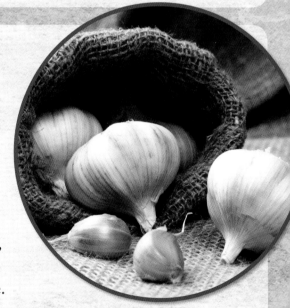

Both the Amish and the Seventh Day Adventists, two religious groups that advocate natural remedies, suggest sucking on a garlic lozenge to treat a sore throat. Garlic, when sliced or crushed, releases the antimicrobial substance allicin. Allicin kills many bacteria, including strep, and some viruses. Seventh Day Adventists Agatha Thrash, M.D., and Calvin Thrash, M.D., in their book *Home Remedies: Hydrotherapy, Massage, Charcoal, and Other Simple Treatments*, say that sore throats sometimes disappear within a few hours of using this technique.

Directions: Slice a garlic clove down the middle and place a half clove on each side of the mouth, between the teeth and cheeks. Suck on the cloves like lozenges as often as necessary.sometimes disappear within a few hours of using this technique.